Epidemiological Research

O.S. Miettinen • I. Karp

Epidemiological Research:
An Introduction

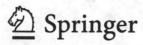
Springer

O.S. Miettinen
McGill University
Université de Montréal
Montréal, QC
Canada

Cornell University
New York, NY
USA

I. Karp
Université de Montréal
Montréal, QC
Canada

ISBN 978-94-017-8411-5   ISBN 978-94-007-4537-7 (eBook)
DOI 10.1007/978-94-007-4537-7
Springer Dordrecht Heidelberg New York London

Printed on acid-free paper

Springer is part of Springer Science+Business Media (www.springer.com)

Foreword

'In my life ever since medical-school graduation half-a-century ago, I've had the dream of reaching true understanding of the theory of the research that would best serve to advance the knowledge-base of medicine, of genuinely scientific medicine.' Olli Miettinen wrote this a year or so ago in his *Epidemiological Research: Terms and Concepts*. For those who have had the privilege to witness his odyssey since the 1970s, the current book comes as both a wonderful revisit of the past and a great leap into the future. Miettinen's text accompanying his course in the 1970s at Harvard was 'the first systematic introduction to theoretical epidemiology' (Greenland) and can be viewed as the start of 'modern epidemiology' (Morabia). But he never published it and therefore the book that you read now is the first published introduction to epidemiological research by the father and grand master of modern epidemiology.

Epidemiological Research: An Introduction, the current book of Miettinen, in collaboration with his junior colleague Igor Karp, is a true milestone for epidemiology, but a cautionary word may be in place about the 'introduction.' I remember Miettinen referring to his courses as basic, but not basal. The current book, similarly, is basic, but not basal. It is introductory in that it develops the objects and methods of epidemiological research from first principles, but it does so in a breathtakingly sophisticated way, alternatingly grand and subtle in argumentation, visionary and down-to-earth, broad and deep. For this reader one thing is particularly clear: Miettinen's discussion is still unparalleled in our field, the logic and coherence is as spellbinding as ever (and I need to think a bit more, and better, if and when I do not fully understand what he writes).

The structure of this book must be a treat for all epidemiologists. From 'epidemiology: grappling with the concept' through 'etiology as a pragmatic concern' and the 'object of study' to the book's core on 'objects design' and 'methods design,' it is like travelling to familiar destinations along new roads. Although Miettinen has always stressed the importance of objects design from first principles, I think this book is the first to treat this topic systematically and somewhat extensively. And although Miettinen has published quite comprehensively on the fallacies in the design of epidemiological studies and their remedies, I find his discussion of 'the etiologic study' fresh and summarized aptly and succinctly in *'e pluribus unum'* and *'e unum pluribus.'*

What will be the effect on the practice of epidemiological research? I have no doubt that it will be vast, but also that it will be slow to come. In the long run, his arguments will turn out to be irresistible, although most likely modified and expanded. It is like the effect of epidemiological research on medical practice: it is hardly ever direct, it nearly always takes a long time, but in the end it makes a true core contribution.

I pay tribute to the father of modern epidemiology, and recommend this volume to assist in deep epidemiological introspection. It will benefit epidemiology and epidemiologists greatly.

Albert Hofman, M.D., Ph.D., Professor and Chair, Department of Epidemiology, Erasmus Medical Center, Rotterdam, The Netherlands.

Preface

Anyone conducting epidemiological research is prone to encounter obvious major challenges of a conceptual nature, sometimes seeing them to be tauntingly complex, at other times subtle beyond concrete grasp. But the challenges can also remain unrecognized and thereby unmet, ones of major consequence included.

Even when no longer a beginner in the research, the investigator may wonder about the adequacy of the copings with these challenges, notably when considering how controversial many of even the much-researched substantive issues remain and, thus, how little consequence the research – his/her own and that of others too – is having in the evolution of knowledge-based societal policies about healthcare and in the advancement of public-health practices within their respective policy frameworks.

The key to attaining, and maintaining, the conceptual understandings that form the basis for maximally consequential careers in epidemiological research we take to be *suitable introduction* to – and thereby the attainment of a wholesome outlook in – such research. To this end, authors of introductory textbooks on the research need to try to present basic ideas that are so obviously *well-focused* and so obviously *tenable* that they thereby get to be – even where they aren't yet – commonly agreed upon by the teachers as properly constituting the core content of an introductory course on the research.

In our view, an introductory course on epidemiological research should bring to focus, and give tenable answers to, such orientational, normative questions as: To what pragmatic ends should the research be conducted? What, as for both substance and form, should the population-level research be about? What should be understood to be the necessary, logical nature of those studies themselves on the principal generic types of object of study? What are the main concerns and principles in the optimization of the objects and methods of those studies? and How should the evidence from the studies be transmuted into knowledge about the respective objects of study?

We here make a serious effort, our first, to formulate answers to these, and related, questions for possible incorporation into teachers' efforts to properly introduce their students to the research – specifically, as insinuated above, to epidemiological research that would be maximally consequential and hence personally most gratifying to them, with society at large not only the sponsor but also the correspondingly, if not even more richly, rewarded beneficiary of it.

In this effort we are guided by our belief that a proper introductory course on epidemiological research, like its counterpart on physics for example, conveys *the most advanced insights into the most elementary* – the most appropriately chosen to be the most elementary – component topics within the overall topic; and our aim is to introduce them in a *logical sequence*, for most natural and effective study by the students. A contemporary introductory course on physics teaches, for example, that the formerly common idea of ether as a ubiquitous medium for electric and magnetic forces (à la Maxwell's equations) is now seen to have been a misunderstanding; and a suitably advanced introductory course on epidemiological research now teaches, for example, that the still-common concepts of cohort study and case-control study should already be passé.

There is a story (apocryphal) about the physicist Niels Bohr and the philosopher Bertrand Russell concerning their respective decisions not to study psychology in preparation for a career in it, about their respective decisions to study mathematics-cum-physics and mathematics-cum-philosophy instead. Bohr is said to have rejected the psychology option on the ground that this field is too easy, and Russell on the ground that it is too difficult, to gain mastery of. We are of the view that preparation for a productive and thereby gratifying career in epidemiological research – different from a stellar career in quantum physics or theoretical philosophy – does not require any extraordinary talent. But we also are keenly aware, from our personal struggles, that it requires *much effort* and – to say it again – a proper introduction and its consequent proper orientation as important prerequisites. The student needs to make the investment of the effort, upon us having endeavored to help the teacher to provide the latter.

Much of an introductory course on epidemiological research necessarily is about *concepts* – and the corresponding terms – germane to such research (refs. 1, 2 below). It thus likely would materially enhance the teaching, and the learning, to supplement this textbook (or any other, for that matter) by a compendium providing suitable introductory exposition and discussion of those concepts and terms (ref. 2), for consultation as needed. For, dwelling on the concepts and terms in the flow of a course like this would tend to take away from the students' grasp of the logic underpinning the sequence of concepts-based *ideas* being introduced, many of them quite original.

References

1. Miettinen OS. Important concepts in epidemiology. In: Olsen J, Saracci R, Trichopoulos D. *Teaching Epidemiology*. Third edition. Oxford: Oxford University Press, 2010.
2. Miettinen OS. *Epidemiological Research: Terms and Concepts*. Dordrecht: Springer, 2011.

Acknowledgements

Miettinen *fils* – a polymath, even if thus far without the evidentiary portfolio of writings – studied a late-version manuscript of this book. We asked him to imagine the youngest one of his children, the only one still young enough to realistically consider, as a potential student of one of this youngster's paternal grandfather's fields (theory of epidemiological research, the other one being theory of meta-epidemiological clinical research) and to consider – critically! – this text as the textbook in that youngster's introduction into this field. And we asked him to comment from the general industrial perspective on what we wrote (sect. 14.5) about epidemiologists' role in quality assurance – economic as well as medical – in the hospital-based segment of healthcare, which in Canada now absorbs about half of the ever less sustainable fiscal burden of the country's public-health industry.

He delighted us, for one, with a learned commentary on introductory teaching of scholarly subjects at large and on how this text conforms with the most notable ideas about it; and for another, he provided us with an equally insightful commentary on industrial quality assurance in general and on its implications for modern public-health practice. And for good measure, he permitted us to incorporate both of these commentaries in this book (Apps. 4, 5).

We also asked Albert Hofman, of Erasmus University Medical Centre, Rotterdam – today's preeminent leader of teaching on all aspects of epidemiological research, from introductory courses on up, in the Erasmus Summer Programme in particular – to critically review a near-final draft of this book, with a view to his possibly writing the Foreword to it.

Hofman indeed was kind enough to read the draft, and he had quite gratifying words to say about it. What is much more, he did agree to write the Foreword. We are much obliged to him.

Contents

Chapter 1
Epidemiology: Grappling with the Concept

Abstract *Public health* as a segment of healthcare naturally is healthcare in the public domain, as distinct from healthcare outside of society's purview; and the care naturally is paramedical care together with medical care – hence the term 'health,' rather than 'medicine,' in 'public health.'

Medicine encompasses *community medicine* in addition to clinical medicine. This segment of medicine inherently is public-health medicine, whereas clinical medicine falls under public health only to the extent that national health insurance has been introduced.

Community medicine used to be focused on *epidemics* of communicable diseases; and a natural term for this segment of medicine thus was *epidemiology*. As the concerns in community medicine were extended to encompass *endemic* occurrence of communicable – and also of non-communicable – illnesses, 'endemiology' could have been introduced as a term for this extension; but instead, the concept of epidemiology was expanded to community medicine in the thus-expanded meaning of it.

Epidemiological research naturally is research to advance (the practice of) community medicine – of epidemiology, that is. This research includes 'bench' or 'basic' research aimed at the development of vaccines, for example; and it falls under various medical sciences instead of constituting a science unto itself.

All of this presumably is natural and quite obviously true in the judgements of beginning students of epidemiological research, but it is here said for the troubling reason that *concepts of epidemiology and epidemiological research different from these are endemic in today's epidemiologic academia.*

The purpose of this chapter is to help the beginning student to find proper orientation in this academia.

O.S. Miettinen and I. Karp, *Epidemiological Research: An Introduction*,
DOI 10.1007/978-94-007-4537-7_1, © Springer Science+Business Media Dordrecht 2012

1.1   Epidemiology as Practice of Healthcare

"The Black Death of 1348 and 1349, and the recurrent epidemics of the fourteenth and fifteenth centuries, were the most devastating natural disasters ever to strike Europe [ref.]. ... Europe about 1420 could have counted barely more than a third of the people it contained one hundred years before." So writes David Herlihy in his *The Black Death and the Transformation of the West* (1997; p. 17).

Herlihy continues: "The devastating plagues elicited a social response that protected the European community from comparable disasters until the present" (p. 17). And: "One hundred years ago, the great bacteriologist Louis Pasteur declared: 'It is now in the power of man to cause all parasitic diseases to disappear from the world' [ref.]" (p. 18).

Regarding Pasteur's grand vision, it is instructive to consider the history of epidemics of smallpox, also known as *variola*.

As there never was any effective treatment for this commonly-fatal communicable disease, healthcare directed to it always focused on *prevention*. Pre-scientifically this was a matter of 'variolation': immunization against variola by means of 'inoculation' (i.e., injection of attenuated matter from variola patients' pustules, to produce a mild case of the disease). Records of this practice in China date back to the sixth century BCE, but in Britain and its American colonies it became rather commonplace only in the early 1700s. While fully effective, it remained controversial on account of concerns about its safety (unintended causation of severe, commonly fatal cases of the disease).

The dawn of science relevant to the practice of variolation was heralded by Benjamin Franklin's work on this. His "goal was simple and straightforward. He wanted to give anxious patients evidence that it was safe to have their children inoculated. The data he assembled were most impressive. ..." This, and more, on Franklin's work on variolation can be found in I. Bernard Cohen's *The Triumph of Numbers: How Counting Changed Modern Life* (2005; p. 90 ff.).

Then came what has been, arguably at least, the most spectacular scientific breakthrough in medicine, resulting in the introduction and adoption of *vaccination* as the replacement of inoculation in the prevention of smallpox. ('Vaccinia' was a synonym for 'cowpox,' the smallpox vaccine being based on matter from pustules of cowpox – a disease similar to but milder than smallpox.) The scientific breakthrough introducing vaccination was not a "triumph of numbers" (cf. above): it resulted from Edward Jenner's work on a single (young) person. But the resulting triumph in medicine was, ultimately, complete: a concerted global program of vaccination, launched by the World Health Organization, resulted in eradication – complete elimination – of the smallpox virus from human populations.

In his *Civilization: The West and the Rest* (2011), Niall Ferguson asserts that "what distinguished the West from the Rest – the mainsprings of global power – were six identifiably novel complexes of institutions and associated ideas and behaviours" (p. 12). One of these he specifies (p. 13) as:

Medicine – a branch of science that allowed a major improvement in health and life expectancy, beginning in Western societies, but also in their colonies

A historiographer as he is, Ferguson is to be forgiven for this excessive deference to medical sources, which commonly (and intentionally?) confuse physicians' practice of healthcare – which we take to be the true concept of medicine – with medical science. "Major improvement" in Western and other societies from practices based on medical science is, however, an incontrovertible fact of history.

Ferguson addresses both medical science and the practice of medicine only in reference to that segment of medicine which produced the historically so consequential, major improvements in human health, namely *community medicine*. For this segment of medicine he uses its umbrella term *'public health,'* which means healthcare in the public domain, and subsumes also paramedical care. He sketches the enormous accomplishments of European medical science in providing the basis for highly effective community programs to prevent infectious diseases, tropical and other, and the startling gains in population health that have been achieved by means of those programs.

Neither that science nor those practices does Ferguson characterize as *epidemiological*, nor as *epidemiology*; in fact, neither one of these terms can be found anywhere in that admirably erudite book. Once aware of this, a student in an introductory course on epidemiological research might be driven to ask: Is this an oversight? or, Is it that there indeed is no epidemiology in the meaning of physicians' epidemiological – community-level – *practice of healthcare*, served by epidemiological research, while clinical research obviously is in the service of physicians' practice of clinical healthcare?

Looking for the answer, the student might explore, for example, the websites concerning *Ottawa Public Health*, the agency providing medical and paramedical healthcare for the community/population of Canada's capital city. This agency is constituted and functioning in accordance with the Health Protection and Promotion Act of the province of Ontario, in which Ottawa is located. "The purpose of this Act is to provide for the organization and delivery of public health programs and services, the prevention of the spread of disease and the promotion and protection of the health of the people of Ontario." Among the "Mandatory health programs and services" this Act specifies, quite notably, "Collection and analysis of *epidemiological* data" (italics ours).

Pursuant to this Act, Ottawa Public Health is headed by a Medical Officer of Health, who is a *"physician* with provincially legislated powers to promote and protect the *public's health"* (italics ours). The other personnel of this agency is composed of "specialized teams of health professionals and support staff, including ... physicians, *epidemiologists*, ..." (italics ours).

This agency periodically publishes the *City of Ottawa Health Status Report*. The latest one, from 2006 (as of Dec. 2011), presents "a wide range of health-related information on mortality, morbidity, communicable diseases, reproductive outcomes, environmental indicators, and behavioral risk factors." It deserves note, in the present context, that of this report's four authors (under the direction and guidance of the Medical Officer of Health), three are specified to be *epidemiologists* – as might be wholly unsurprising, given what the report is about. And let's be clear: they are not reporting on epidemiological research (scientific) but on their *practice as epidemiologists*.

It thus is evident that epidemiology in at least one meaning of the term is community medicine, practice of this. In fact, this could well be the only meaning of the term: Research for clinical medicine is termed clinical research; but this research is not thought of as constituting one of the meanings – much less the only meaning – of 'clinical medicine.' By analogy, it would seem natural to think of epidemiological research as being extrinsic to that which it serves, namely epidemiology in the meaning of community medicine, its practice; it would seem natural to think that the research is not epidemiology by virtue of being in service of epidemiology. In these terms, just as a clinical researcher is not inherently a clinician, so an epidemiological researcher is not inherently an epidemiologist.

The work of Ottawa Public Health illustrates the essence of epidemiology as a genre of the practice of healthcare: not only is it community medicine but, as such, it inherently is (a physician's practice of) *public health* as a matter of *community-level preventive medicine*. More on this in the last chapter (ch. 14) of this book.

Eminent in public-health practices in respect to non-communicable diseases have been those centering on *occupational* populations. As Robert Proctor points out in his *The Nazi War on Cancer* (1999), "German physicians had a long tradition in industrial hygiene, and Nazi physicians continued this practice"; and the very major anti-cancer program of that era (1933–1945) in Germany had an "emphasis on occupational carcinogenesis" (p. 73).

In a 1973 book entitled *Occupational Health Practice*, M.L. Newhouse and R.S.F. Schilling (the Editor) have a chapter on "Uses and methods of epidemiology." They say that for an occupational health service "to achieve higher standards of health in a working community, it is essential to observe people as groups by using the methods of epidemiology, 'a branch of medical science ... '" (p. 169). To them – and by no means alone – occupational-health practice is not practice of epidemiology but, instead, involves *use* of it, of the methods of that "science." They refer to a textbook source with a telling title: *Uses of Epidemiology* (Morris JN, 1964).

The physicians who, in Ottawa and elsewhere, produced the community diagnoses about, say, the SARS and H1N1 ('swine flu') epidemics and directed the population-level programs to control these, and physicians who are caring for, say, occupational populations as populations (rather than individually), we really think of as epidemiologists in the practice of epidemiology – of community-medicine, that is. We really do not think of them as 'users' of epidemiology in something that is not epidemiology.

1.2 Epidemiology as Health Research

Oncology, in one meaning of the term, is a discipline ('specialty') of medicine; it is the discipline of a physician's practice of cancer-related healthcare, clinical or community-level practice. Oncology also is a science; it is the medical science aimed at advancing the practice of oncology. Oncological research is 'applied' science in this meaning; and this it is regardless of how 'basic' it is – as when aimed at, say, potential development of a proteomic 'biomarker' for latent-stage diagnoses about a cancer or a protein to 'turn off' an activated proto-oncogene in the treatment of a cancer.

By analogy, this: Insofar as the practice of community medicine is viewed as being epidemiology, *epidemiological research* is naturally taken to be research – *any* research, however 'basic' – aimed at advancement of the practice of community medicine. We hold to the predicate in this (sect. 1.1 above), and we therefore hold this inclusive conception of epidemiological research.

The earliest, and arguably the most spectacular, example of epidemiological research, in these terms, is the study for which Edward Jenner is so famous (sect. 1.1). He injected into a little boy, who had not experienced smallpox, matter from a cowpox lesion of someone else; and when Jenner a few weeks later inoculated this boy with smallpox matter, the boy did not come down with smallpox – the boy evidently had been immunized against this much more serious disease. (Jenner had developed, as a practitioner, the impression that those having undergone cowpox had been resistant to smallpox.) And recent examples include, among others, the research culminating in the availability of a vaccine for the prevention of HPV infection and, thereby, prevention of cervical cancer.

The concepts of oncological and epidemiological research are not fully analogous, however. Oncological research in the aggregate amounts to a science (called oncology), in the research (rather than knowledge) meaning of that science. This is because oncological research has a coherent, singular subject-matter or 'material object,' namely malignant neoplasm. Epidemiological research, very different from this, can address a material object from any one of a large number of health sciences – oncology, immunology (as in Jenner's case), etc. As a consequence, *epidemiological research is not definitional to a science* (called epidemiology); it – like morphological research, for example – is subsumed under a variety of sciences.

Students of epidemiological research are prone to be left confused about the essence of this line of research, at least early in their studies. To wit, one of us wrote his thesis for the degree of Master of Public Health, in 1964, on *Epidemiology and Its Method*, which at the time were topics of vigorous debate in the *American Journal of Public Health*. Drawing from the various then-prevailing definitions, he merely synthesized them – in the framework of explicit principles – as amounting to this: "Epidemiology is the science of the occurrence of health and illness; the scope of epidemiology is the entirety of the occurrence of health and illness; and the method of epidemiology is essentially the scientific method but may have some distinctive characteristics." He thus found, most notably, that to his elders epidemiology was a *science*, and only this, rather than the practice of community medicine, this alone (cf. Schilling in sect. 1.1). He refrained from expressing his own views about these ideas of his elders (even though he hadn't been brought up in the Presbyterian culture).

David Lilienfeld – son of the eminent epidemiologist Abraham Lilienfeld – when he still was a college student in the 1970s, took a more-than-casual interest in what his father's field really was. He delved deep into the literature on the matter; and he brought to view 23 published definitions of epidemiology, the first one from 1927. Dissatisfied with them all, he added one of his own: epidemiology is "a method of reasoning about disease that deals with biological inferences derived from observations of disease phenomena in population groups." (The culture surrounding his youthful development – different from that of the youngster alluded to above – presumably was the one which, quite uniquely, encourages *critical* study of the Scripture, even.)

We present, in Table 1.1 below, seven notable definitions of epidemiology, from 1956 to the present. The strong impression from these definitions, disappointing to us, is that epidemiology is seen to be a matter of research alone, and this, even, without any inherent service relation to the practice of healthcare – different from, say, that of oncological research in relation to the practice of oncology (cf. above). It seems that the research is seen to be conducted for the sake of the research itself, as though there were no practice of epidemiology being served by the research (cf. sect. 1.1).

It really does seem, on the basis of those definitions, that among epidemiological researchers of late there hasn't been any conception of epidemiology as practice of healthcare. Sight seems to have been lost of the field pioneered by Hippocrates pre-scientifically, as most notably described in his *Of the Epidemics*; this field made vastly more consequential by the spectacular scientific contributions to it by Edward Jenner, John Snow, Louis Pasteur, and Robert Koch, among others; this field later extended to combating also epidemics of non-communicable illnesses such as congenital malformations, cancers, degenerative cardiovascular diseases, and diabetes; this field now combating even endemic rates of population occurrence of whatever type of illness. These practices do exist (sect. 1.1), and they are very important. But these practices of community medicine, according to the definitions in Table 1.1, are not epidemiology; and Ottawa Public Health, when it periodically reports on the health of the city's residents, as determined in its practices there, is not, according to those definitions, reporting on epidemiology. (Cf. sect. 1.1.)

According to most of those definitions in Table 1.1, epidemiology is merely the '*study*' of something, sometimes alternatively (and unjustifiably; cf. above) said to be the '*science*' of that something; and to this has recently – and only exceptionally – been added application of the results of that study. We take those definitions to be intended to mean that epidemiology is, in the only meaning of the term, a line of *research* – population-level research on the rates of occurrence of phenomena of human health.

In those definitions there is no expression of the conception of a certain type of practice of healthcare as inherently being epidemiology, even when its knowledge-base does not derive from epidemiology-the-study. The knowledge-base

Table 1.1   Select definitions of epidemiology

Maxcy KF. Epidemiology. In: Maxcy KF (Editor). *Rosenau Preventive Medicine and Public Health*. 8th edition. New York: Appleton-Century-Crofts, 1956:

> "that field of medical science which is concerned with the relationships of the various factors and conditions that determine the frequencies and distributions of an infectious process, a disease, or a physiological state in a human community" (p.1289)

MacMahon B, Pugh TF, Ipsen J. *Epidemiologic Methods*. Boston: Little, Brown and Company, 1960:

> "the study of the distribution and determinants of disease prevalence in man" (p.3)

Lilienfeld AM. *Foundations of Epidemiology*. New York: Oxford University Press, 1976:

> "the study of the distribution of a disease or a physiological condition in human populations and of the factors that influence this distribution" (p. 3)

Sartwell PE, Last JM. Epidemiology. In: Last JM (Editor). *Maxcy-Rosenau Preventive Medicine and Public Health*. 11th edition. New York: Appleton-Century-Crofts, 1980:

> "the study of the distribution and dynamics of disease in populations" (p. 9)

Last JM (Editor). *A Dictionary of Epidemiology*. 1st edition. Oxford: Oxford University Press, 1983:

> "the study of the distribution and determinants of health-related states and events in populations, and the application of this study to control of health problems"

Rothman KJ, Greenland S, Lash TL. *Modern Epidemiology*. 3rd edition. Philadelphia: Lippincott Williams & Wilkins, 2008:

> "the study of the distribution of health-related states and events in populations" (p. 32)

Porta M (Editor), Greenland S, Last JM (Associate Editors). *A Dictionary of Epidemiology*. 5th edition. Oxford: Oxford University Press, 2008:

> "the study of the occurrence and distribution of health-related states or events in specified populations, including the study of the determinants influencing such states, and the application of this knowledge to control the health problems"

of 'mass' screening for tuberculosis has been entirely clinical and, thus, not even in part the result of epidemiological "study." Such screening therefore has not been epidemiology according to any of those definitions. Nor were the recent population-level efforts to control the SARS and H1N1 ('swine flu') epidemics epidemiology, as they were programs of the practice, not ones of mere *"study."*

With academics having lost sight of epidemiology as practice of healthcare (of community-level preventive medicine), epidemiological research does not get to be defined according to what it is intended to serve. It used to be commonly defined by the use of 'the epidemiological method' (cf. above), but more recently it is commonly defined in terms of something about its objects of study. And whereas all phenomena of health are in its purview, as potential material objects of the research, the felt need now is to define epidemiological research by its formal objects, the (characteristic) *form* of its objects (on whatever phenomena of health). This is what the definitions in that Table 1.1 are about.

However well this is done, the implication is that excluded from epidemiological research is the 'basic' or 'bench' research that underpins, for example, the development of vaccines. In these terms – by the form of its objects – one can define only a part of what we take to be epidemiological research (cf. above). This, we hold, should be the idea. For by no means is all of the research relevant to dealing with communicable-disease epidemics, for example, singular in the form of its objects, just as, say, oncological research isn't.

Insofar as there is taken to be a definitional form of the objects of epidemiological research, this has to do with research on phenomena of health on the population – 'mass' – level, the level of community medicine. Relative to the clinical level, phenomena of health on this higher level have new, 'emergent' properties. On the clinical level a given phenomenon of health characterizes an individual at a particular moment in time; the phenomenon either is or is not associated with that person-moment; it either is or is not occurring in it; it has no frequency of occurrence at that person-moment. On the population level, by contrast, any given phenomenon of health inherently occurs, and doesn't occur, in association with a multitude of person-moments. It has, thus, the emergent quality of the frequency – the *rate* – of this occurrence. This is the central element in the form of the objects in epidemiological research on the population (rather than 'bench') level.

A health phenomenon's rate of occurrence (on the population level) is, inherently, a *quantitative* phenomenon; but the rate quite generally is non-singular in magnitude. Its level varies according to various *determinants* of this level; it is a *function* of its determinants. Therefore, epidemiological research, when addressing rates of occurrence of phenomena of health, necessarily has *occurrence relations* as its objects: a health phenomenon's rate of occurrence in relation to – as a function of – its determinants, this in a defined *domain* of people.

Given those definitions in Table 1.1 above, it should be noted that population-level epidemiological research is *not* about the "distributions" of the phenomena of health; and that the determinants of the rates of occurrence of phenomena of health are *not* objects of epidemiological research – only rates' relations to these are. On the clinical level, cases of a phenomenon of health inherently have a distribution by gender and age, for example, while on the population level the phenomenon has a rate of occurrence that may, or may not, depend on gender and age. And, for example, behavioral determinants of the occurrence of phenomena of health are objects of study in behavioral and social sciences and not in epidemiological research, which is biomedical science (though not constituting a science; cf. above).

1.3 Epidemiology as a Research Discipline

There is no single discipline of how to conduct oncological research – no textbooks nor any 'training' courses on what, as to form at least, to study and how. In 'basic' oncological research in particular, progress is not a consequence of professionalism in the research. Instead, progress derives from the process of creative conjectures and their critical testings, as the philosopher Karl Popper explains in his venerable *Conjectures and Refutations* (1963). In these terms there may be no limits to scientific progress, as the polymath David Deutsch argues in his *The Beginning of Infinity* (2011). A wonderful "biography" of oncological research is *The Emperor of All Maladies* (2010) by Siddharta Mukherjee.

When a line of health research is defined by the *form* of its objects, without coherence of the material objects, as epidemiological research now commonly is (sect. 1.2 above), there is a corresponding opportunity together with, as usual, a corresponding risk. That the focus in this research is on objects of a singular form – that of occurrence relations (sect. 1.2) – provides for the development of a more-or-less coherent body of theory to guide research on objects of that form, a learnable *research discipline* for professional study of phenomena of health on the population level – and of non-health phenomena just the same. An associated risk is a certain *formalism* in the research – replacement of creative and critical thought by mere conformity with the prevailing professional norms, unjustifiable ones included.

The discipline of how to conduct population-level health research is the subject of several contemporary textbooks of "Epidemiology" (e.g., MacMahon and Trichopoulos, 1996, and Rothman et alii, 2008), implying that this discipline is the denotation – the only one – of 'epidemiology.' To us this is, however, only one – the most recent, a third – meaning of the term (cf. sects. 1.1, 1.2), and a questionable one at that.

The Enlightenment maxim *Sapere aude!* ('Dare to reason!'), eminently propagated by the philosopher Immanuel Kant among others, should be understood to apply to the prevailing teachings about epidemiological occurrence research as well. After all, questioning received knowledge (scholastic) was at the very core of Enlightenment; and the Enlightenment outlook in turn was the springboard of the enormous progress in science subsequent to the advent of this outlook in the seventeenth century, as Ferguson explains (sect. 1.1) – even if, arguably at least, its antecedent scientific progress was at the root of Enlightenment. (In the pre-Enlightenment era, Copernicus dared publish only post-humously, while Galileo was more courageous than that and suffered for it.)

When people in our 'post-industrial' societies concern themselves with that which is the concern in community medicine – in epidemiology in this meaning of population-level practice of preventive healthcare (sect. 1.1) – they think of their *nutrition* – diet and dietary supplements – first and foremost. It therefore is particularly illustrative of epidemiological research in this disciplinary sense of it, to examine its accomplishments with focus on nutrition: what is known? what is the basis of this knowledge from epidemiological research? and what does this say about the scientific prowess of our contemporary discipline of epidemiological research?

We devote much of chapter 2 of this book to this topic. It illustrates the stagnation that in research tends to flow from formalism – and from its associated academic routine of counting publications instead of contributions. The *central flaw* in today's disciplinary framework of epidemiological research is, as we will illustrate, its focus on the methodology of the research, without regard for disciplined *objects design* before methods design. (Stagnation consequent to formalism in societal development was a major concern of the Soviet leader Michael Gorbachev when he launched his famous programs of openness/*glasnost* and restructuring/*perestroika*.)

1.4   Epidemiology as a Subject of Study

As set forth in the three sections above, there now is epidemiology in three different meanings of the term; and there could just as well be a fourth one: given that there is epidemiology in the meaning of the theory – concepts and principles (and terminology) – of epidemiological research (sect. 1.3 above), a related, more proximal but very different meaning of 'epidemiology' would be that of the theory of epidemiological practice, a theoretical discipline yet to be introduced, even though that of clinical practice has been – in *Up from Clinical Epidemiology & EBM* (2011) by one of us.

Given the prevailing triad of meanings of 'epidemiology' (sects. 1.1, 1.2, 1.3 above), a student now pursuing an academic degree in epidemiology unspecified (as now is usual) needs to be clear on which one of the prevailing three meanings of the term is the one of his/her chosen future career. For this is a prerequisite for understanding how the studies preparatory to the career should be composed from the three epidemiologies that now may be available for study.

As for epidemiology in the meaning of a *discipline of research*, the most important orientational questions are these: Does a future practitioner of community medicine need to study this? and, To what extent does study of this discipline constitute the necessary preparation for a career in epidemiological research? To that first question our answer is simple: Not really, but an introductory course might be a justifiable investment of time and effort, with merely impressionistic education the aim of this. (The future practitioner really would need to study the theory – concepts and principles – of the practice, were such study to be available, and then the current knowledge-base of this practice and how to update this knowledge.) And to that second question our answer, below, is rather involved. Preparation for a career on the theory of population-level epidemiological research – the development and teaching of this – is a very uncommon concern of the student, and it thus is not our express concern in this book, even though an introductory course on epidemiological research is very useful for the future theoretician as well.

The student whose future career will be one of population-level epidemiological research needs to make good choices in relevant areas. One of these – now receiving much too little attention – has to do with the substantive focus in the studies, including in any thesis work (of which the subsequent research commonly is an unwitting extension). For (s)he needs to understand that society does not sponsor the research in order that the researchers can indulge in their interests; there needs to be a societally justifiable purpose in the research (cf. Preface). Consider two examples:

One of us, as a doctoral student of epidemiology, half-a-century ago, thought that a good topic for his PhD thesis in epidemiology would be the rate of biological ageing, this in causal relation to various aspects of lifestyle. In fact, he thought that this would be a good line of research for his entire career, and for a number of other researchers as well. These judgements sprang from his consideration of the public's great concern to retard the process together with his vision of the feasibility of studying it – feasibility critically in terms of how an operational scale for the rate of ageing could be developed. He therefore studied, on his own and in depth, the biology of ageing. But in the end he did not pursue this research, because he judged that his preordained career line, one in that prevailing third meaning of 'epidemiology' – before extending it to the theory of clinical research – is better served by further studies in 'biostatistics' and thesis work in this area. (This judgement he did implement.)

Another example to consider is the entire realm of 'social epidemiology,' now in notable ascendancy. In it, the concern is to study population health in relation – causal relation – to such 'social' characterizers of people as their race and level of income, for example. But for health effects of race to represent even a theoretically admissible choice – let alone a good one – for epidemiological research, it should be that race effects on health (or whatever else) are imaginable; but they aren't, given that for a person's actual race there was no alternative: a given, real person could not have been conceived and born as a representative of some alternative race; for a given person the racial implication of the pair of parental gametes is an immutable given. And if it be granted – even if only for the sake of argument – that the relative effects of alterative distributions of income on population health are meaningfully studyable, meaningful questions would arise. For example: Would this research possibly help justify societal policies concerning, say, minimum wage? Would it even be considered? Or is it, instead, that poverty is, and is to be viewed as, a problem as such, and not because of what it causes as health effects, for example. More on this in section 2.6.

A student preparing for a career in epidemiological research should enter into a career-long program of self-development with a view to maximizing good choices for the substantive topics of his/her research. Central to this pursuit is understanding what the best source of advice is, namely, the practitioners out there. So, if the student would contemplate, and have difficulty perceiving, the relative merits of the two lines of research in the examples above, (s)he should ask epidemiologists of the first – practicing – type (sect. 1.1) this: For you to better serve the protection of your client population's health, which one of these two would you rather learn from epidemiological research: the effects of carbohydrate-rich diets on individuals' rates of biological ageing, or the health effects of low wages?

Thus, a student preparing for a career in community-level health research (biomedical; sects. 1.2, 2.6) needs to get to the habit – career-long habit – of maintaining up-to-date familiarity with the goings-on in the practice of community medicine, notably with a view to familiarity with the *gaps in the knowledge-base of the practices* as seen by the practitioners themselves. The academic program should include arrangements for the students' inquisitive mingling with practitioners.

Parallel with this program of maintaining awareness of the goings-on in the 'field' there is, of course, the need for a counterpart of this in respect to epidemiological research, which, ideally at least, is in the service of the practice. The research at large deserves only superficial following, to remain up-to-date on what the topics are. On the other hand, research in one's own area of subject-matter needs to be followed both inclusively and in depth, the relevant 'basic' research included.

No good purpose in the education of epidemiological researchers, we think, is served by a general course addressing research on select topics in 'substantive epidemiology,' given the great diversity of subject-matter in the students' future lines of epidemiological research – or, for that matter, of epidemiological-type research that actually is extraepidemiological. Equally meaningless are seminar presentations of studies on a limitless mélange of subject-matter, empty of content that the audience at large should consider for self-development as epidemiological researchers.

Last, but by no means least, the most obvious point here: For future researchers on population-level topics of the epidemiological form (as superficially specified in sect. 1.3 above) the generally directly-relevant preparatory studies toward good choices are ones of the *theory* of that research. Epidemiology in this research-discipline sense is what the studies principally are about. Study of it should be materially – indeed, critically – helpful in efforts to optimize decisions about what, exactly, to study – a matter of the studies' objects design – and also how to study it – a matter of the studies' methods design – so long as at issue is population-level (rather than 'basic') research.

It may not be obvious, however, what these theory studies, even in their broadest outlines, are or should be about. But even before this question there is the one about the necessary *prerequisites* for these studies. The student should master certain general concepts of medicine and science, but the availability of a suitable reference text should allow inquiry into these as needed, rather than necessarily in advance of the studies on the theory specific to population-level epidemiological research. (Cf. Preface.)

The student absolutely needs a background in (probability theory and then) *statistics*. For as mathematics is to physics, so statistics is to population-level epidemiological research. Major background study of mathematics is an absolute prerequisite for any serious study for a career in physics; but: mathematics is not the theory – the embodiment of the concepts and principles – of physics, nor is physics an outgrowth of mathematics (a field of meta-mathematics, as it were). The objects of population-level epidemiological research are generally about frequencies (sect. 1.2) and hence statistical in form; such epidemiological research therefore is statistical research in form (while medical in substance). But as with mathematics in relation physics, *statistics is not, nor does it subsume, the theory of population-level epidemiological research.*

Students of epidemiological research thus need to have suitable preparatory education in (probability theory and) statistics, and of course the necessary mathematical preparedness for this. The suitable education in statistics would mainly focus on topics of 'multiple regression'; and it would not confuse and mislead the students with endogenously statistical ideas about research – with 'survey research,' 'sample size determination,' 'multiple hypothesis testing,' and 'data-suggested hypotheses,' among others. For, to say it again, statistics is not, nor does it subsume, the theory of statistical science.

The rest of this book is, in the main, quite extensive an exposition of what we think these theory studies should be about, on the introductory level. But in utterly succinct terms, as insinuated above, it can be said that at issue really are only two broad topics: *objects design* and *methods design* for population-level epidemiological research. With these broad topics suitably construed, theory of epidemiological 'data analysis' (really, synthesis of the data to the study result) becomes essentially a non-topic.

As a student setting out to prepare for a career in epidemiological research grapples with the concept of epidemiology per se and that of epidemiological research in relation to this – these frustrating topics at the very outset of the studies – (s)he would do well, we think, being mindful of two principles bearing on this.

1. Critical for progress in any field of science generally is propitious definition of the field in question. Highly illustrative of this is the historical fact that chemistry started its spectacular progress only once Robert Boyle distinguished between mixtures and compounds; defined elements as constituents of compounds, introducing the term 'analysis' for the study of these compositions (cf. 'data analysis' as a term for data synthesis, above); and defined chemistry itself by its being not about mixtures but about compounds. These 'revolutionary' ideas he set forth in his book fittingly entitled *The Sceptical Chymist* (1661).

   The student of epidemiological research should reflect on the relative merits of defining epidemiological research as (*a*) the study of the distribution and determinants of phenomena of health in human populations (or some variant of this), or as (*b*) research – including 'basic' research – for advancement of the practice of community medicine, of epidemiology in this meaning.

2. "Read not to contradict, nor to believe, but to weigh and consider" (ref. 1 below). In his/her understanding of the theory of epidemiological research, the student of this will ultimately be alone, solely responsible for his/her own (*sic*) understanding. "For the vision of one man lends not its wings to another man" (ref. 2 below). (A practitioner of epidemiology, by contrast, needs to defer to experts' shared beliefs – knowledge in this meaning – on the substantive topics that are relevant.)

References

1. Bacon F. Of studies. *In*: Bacon F. *The Essays or Counsels Civil and Moral*. Edited with an Introduction and Notes by Brian Vickers. Oxford: Oxford University Press, 1999; p. 134.
2. Gibran K. On teaching. *In*: Gibran K. *The Prophet*. New York: Alfred A Knopf, 1970.

Chapter 2
Epidemiological Knowledge: Examples

Abstract Whereas the natural – the only justifiable – purpose of epidemiological research is the advancement of epidemiology in the meaning of (the practice of) community medicine, a student starting to prepare for epidemiological research naturally wishes to gain some orientational sense of the status of *knowledge* – and then, especially, of lack thereof – relevant to community medicine, despite the vastness of the number of issues involved in this. In respect to the status of the knowledge there thus is a need for suitable focusing of the exploration.

One guide to the selection of a suitable focus in the exploration of the present state of epidemiological knowledge is the fact that community medicine is *preventive* – rather than curative/therapeutic or rehabilitative – medicine. The knowledge-base of community medicine thus is naturally organized by *determinants* (causal) of population health, with a view to all of the various health implications of these – rather than by health outcomes, with prevention of each treated as separate topics. Thus, an encyclopedia of preventive medicine would address the entirety of the health effects of smoking under the rubric of smoking – not the role of smoking in the causation of various illnesses, with these outcomes as the organizing principle.

In this spirit, we focus on the eminent topic of *nutrition* as a determinant of select aspects of health. More specifically, we mainly address the fats-versus-carbohydrates contrast in the energy content of the diet, but to an extent we also address omega-3 fatty acids, antioxidants, and salt in the diet.

As another, very different depiction of the state of epidemiological knowledge (concerning the prevention of illness) we examine the annual issues of *Epidemiologic Reviews*, representing the state of the art – these reviews being "comprehensive and critical" and produced under the auspices of an eminent school of public health together with an eminent journal of "epidemiology" affiliated with it.

O.S. Miettinen and I. Karp, *Epidemiological Research: An Introduction,*
DOI 10.1007/978-94-007-4537-7_2, © Springer Science+Business Media Dordrecht 2012

2.1   Nutrition and Atherogenesis

In epidemiological practice (of community medicine; sect. 1.1), an eminent line of action is population-level *health education*, and especially that about lifestyles – education that presumedly is based on professional knowledge about the health consequences of various features of lifestyle when maintained in lieu of particular alternatives to these. The regulatory and service approaches to improvement of population health are, of course, equally dependent on the availability of knowledge of what in people's lives bears on the preservation of their health, and to what extent. The relevant knowledge is about health in relation (causal) to lifestyles in respect to nutrition first and foremost.

Among people's common nutrition-related health concerns are the risks of 'degenerative' vascular diseases (mostly coronary and cerebro-vascular disease) consequent to relatively advanced stages of *atheromatosis* (fatty deposits in arteries; Gr. *athērē*, 'gruel'). And nutrition-based prevention of these diseases therefore is principally directed to slowing down the process (life-long) of the progression of atheromatosis – of further *atherogenesis*, that is. (Thrombogenesis is a related other concern, though much less eminent; Gr. *thrombos*, 'clot.')

Concerning the present state of knowledge about the role of nutrition in atherogenesis, there scarcely is an exposition superior to *Good Calories, Bad Calories: Fats, Carbs, and the Controversial Science of Diet and Health* (2007), by Gary Taubes. The title is telling: the science concerned with something that is of central concern in community-level preventive medicine – and in its clinical counterpart too – remains a matter of eminent controversies. In fact, so Taubes argues, the now-dominant central tenets about nutritional atherogenesis are likely wrong. In developing his ideas he draws from epidemiological research in the inclusive meaning we give to this, 'basic' research very definitely included (sect. 1.2).

Taubes focuses on the relative proportions of fats and carbohydrates in the overall energy composition of diet, fully appreciating that a low-fat diet tends to be, in isocaloric terms, a diet correspondingly high in carbohydrates, and conversely. Related to this, in his book, "Part I is entitled 'The Fat-Cholesterol Hypothesis' and describes how we came to believe that heart disease is caused by the effect of dietary fat and particularly saturated fat on the cholesterol in our blood. It evaluates the evidence to support that hypothesis. Part II is entitled 'The Carbohydrate Hypothesis.' It describes the history of the carbohydrate hypothesis of chronic disease, beginning in the nineteenth century. It then discusses in some detail the science that has evolved since the 1960s to support this hypothesis, and how this evidence was interpreted once public-health authorities established the fat-cholesterol hypothesis as conventional wisdom" (p. xxiii).

While Parts I and II indeed evaluate those profoundly different hypotheses, a much larger picture actually is painted by the two: how the purported knowledge about the role of diet in atherogenesis, as formulated by health agencies – both non-governmental and governmental – and even by a committee of the U.S. Senate, is a consequence of the superficial appeal of the now-dominant hypothesis (postulating an atherogenetic effect of dietary fat, mediated by level of serum cholesterol); the zealous and persistent campaign of the originator of that hypothesis (Ancel Keys) and of his adherents (Jeremiah Stamler, i.a.) to keep that hypothesis alive; and various improprieties that have distorted the translation of the evidence into purported knowledge.

Following some laboratory experiments on animals of arguably misleading (herbivorous) species, the initial human-level evidence for the fat-cholesterol conception of atherogenesis was derived from geographic comparisons (by Keys); but it was, as Taubes explains, biased by design. On the other hand, evidence against it – commonly ignored – came from the venerable Framingham Heart Study – even if an important part of this the proponents of the hypothesis kept unpublished for a long time. Countervailing evidence from a randomized trial by partisans of that conception also was substantially delayed in its publication.

Regarding the carbohydrate hypothesis, Taubes describes, extensively, "the science that was pushed aside as investigators and public-health authorities tried to convince first themselves and then the rest of us that dietary fat was the root of all nutritional evils" (p. 152). The pushed-aside science at issue here concerns, most eminently, two topics: blood levels of triglycerides and lipoproteins and their dependence on carbohydrates rather than saturated fats in the diet; and the 'saccharine disease' or 'syndrome x' or *metabolic syndrome* conception of 'diseases of civilization,' coronary heart disease among these, with dietary carbohydrates – refined starches and sugar in particular – the 'civilized' cause of this aggregate of diseases.

This pushed-aside science is, as Taubes describes it, complex but quite compelling. All of it is epidemiological in our inclusive meaning of 'epidemiological research,' though largely not in the now-common, restricted meaning (sect. 1.2). As public-health science, when all of its 'chronic-disease' implications are considered, the importance of this nutritional science is second only to the science – epidemiological laboratory science – that provided for 'the ascent of man' (Jacob Bronowski) over the scourges of communicable-disease epidemics (sects. 1.1, 1.2). ('Chronic disease,' while a term in common use by epidemiologists, is not apposite as an antonym of 'communicable disease.')

In the face of all of this, the young student of epidemiological research would do well, we suggest, sharing the optimistic view of the eminent physicist Richard Feynman, whom Taubes quotes as having said that, whatever be one's bias, there comes a time when the "perpetual accumulation of [evidence] ... cannot be discarded any longer" (p. 83).

Another eminent topic in dietary causation – etiology/etiogenesis – of atheromatotic disease now has to do with paucity of *omega-3 fatty acids* in the diet. Taubes does not deal with this, but the two Scientific Statements on this topic by the American Heart Association are of note.

In the first one of these two Statements – Stone JF, *Circulation* 1996; 94: 2337-40 – the up-front content is this: "Reducing intake of saturated fat and dietary cholesterol and avoiding excess calories, which can lead to obesity, remain the cornerstone of the dietary approach to decreasing risk of atherosclerotic vascular disease [cf. above]. During the past 20 years, however, there has been renewed interest in other dietary components that might favorably improve [*sic*] lipid profiles and reduce risk of coronary heart disease (CHD). Fish and fish oil, rich sources of omega-3 fatty acids, have sparked intense interest in both epidemiological studies, which suggest a favorable effect on CHD, and metabolic ward studies, which show a striking improvement in lipid profiles in hyperlipidemic patients. Confusion has resulted from clinical trials of fish oil in patients with CHD, which did not corroborate early observational findings, and newer results, which suggest clinical benefit due to a mechanism independent of lipid effects."

The more recent, second Statement – Krist-Etherton PM et alii, *Circulation* 2002; 106: 2747-57 – has a summary which opens thus: "Omega-3 fatty acids have been shown in epidemiological and clinical trials to reduce the incidence of CVD. Large-scale epidemiological studies suggest that individuals at risk for CHD benefit from the consumption of plant- and marine-derived omega-3 fatty acids, although the ideal intakes presently are unclear." Said in the body of this Statement is that in a recent "meta-analysis" of the results of 11 randomized trials "with 7951 patients in the intervention groups, ... the risk ratio of nonfatal MI was 0.8, for fatal MI it was 0.7, and for sudden death (in 5 trials) it was 0.7" – as though these numbers had meaning without specificity in respect to the actual contrast and its duration, and the domain of this.

So, while popular interest in this nutritional topic also is broadly-based and keen, available from epidemiological research on it seems to be conflictual ideas and meaningless empirical numbers rather than secure knowledge derived from meaningful evidence.

2.2 Nutrition and Oncogenesis

Taubes (ref. in sect. 2.1 above) makes a quite compelling case for *cancer*, too, being a 'disease of civilization,' emerging in all essence only with the advent of the 'civilized' diet – low in fats and high in carbohydrates – as a feature of agricultural societies, up to 10,000 years already.

He describes as a piece of "seminal work" a 120-page report by Richard Doll and Richard Peto, in 1981, "that reviewed the existing evidence on changes in cancer incidence over time, changes upon migration from one region of the world to another, and differences in cancer rates between communities and nations" (p. 209). They concluded, Taubes says, that diet was "causing 35 percent of all cancers, though the uncertainties they considered to be so vast that the number could be as low as 10 percent or as high as 70 percent" (pp. 209-10).

"By the end of the 1990s, clinical trials and large-scale prospective studies had demonstrated that the dietary fat and fiber hypotheses of cancer were almost assuredly wrong, and similar investigations had repeatedly failed to confirm that red meat played any role" (p. 211).

The 'saccharine disease' or 'metabolic syndrome' concept having been advanced decades earlier (cf. sect. 2.1 above), Taubes points out that Richard Doll and Bruce Armstrong "had found sugar intake in international comparisons to be 'positively correlated with both the incidence and mortality from' colon, rectal, breast, ovarian, prostate, kidney, nervous-system, and testicular cancer, and that 'other investigators have produced similar findings'" (pp. 211-2).

Taubes proceeds to an extensive and deep examination of the role, in oncogenesis (Gr. *oncos*, 'mass, bulk'), of two hormones whose blood levels are closely connected to carbohydrates in the diet, namely *insulin* and *insulin-like growth factor* (IGF). That these hormones play a substantial role in both the genesis and growth of cancers, and that therefore dietary carbohydrates do, he makes quite plausible – even if these insights, too, tend to be 'pushed aside' (cf. sect. 2.1 above) by authorities on nutrition and (public) health.

Taubes refers twice to the 700-page report *Food, Nutrition and Prevention of Cancer,* published in 1997 by the World Cancer Research Fund together with the American Institute for Cancer Research. He writes that "the assembled experts could find neither 'convincing' nor even 'probable' reason to believe that fat-rich diets increased the risk of cancer" (p. 74). And as for carbohydrates, he quotes (p. 118) from the report this:

> The degree to which starch is refined in diets, particularly when the intake of starch is high, may itself be an important factor in cancer risk, as may be the volume of refined starches and sugars in diets. Epidemiological studies have not, however, generally distinguished between degrees of refining or processing of starches, and there are, as yet, no reliable epidemiological data on the effects of refining on cancer risk.

The Cancer Prevention Overview (PDQ®) of the U.S. National Cancer Institute, the Health Professional Version of this (consulted in December 2011, last modified 04/29/2011), gives the following synopsis of that massive WCRF/AICR review:

> With respect to dietary factors that may protect against cancer, the greatest consistency was seen for fruits and non-starchy vegetables. In the WCRF/AICR report, conclusions were reached that both fruits and non-starchy vegetables were associated with 'probable decreased risk' of lung cancer. Thus, even for the two dietary exposure classes that the current evidence suggests may have the greatest cancer prevention potential, the evidence was judged to be less than convincing and was applicable to only a few malignancies.

From this it may appear that the WCRF/AICR review had nothing to say about cancer prevention in accordance with either one of the two hypotheses addressed by Taubes – not by avoidance of fats nor by avoidance of carbohydrates, in the diet. These topics are, however, among the 61 (*sic*) items of food and drink the WCRT/AICR report addressed in terms of "total fat" and "foods containing sugars," and neither one of these two did the WCRF/AICR experts judge to confer "convincing increased risk" or "probably increased risk" for any of the 13 cancers (by site; table in the foldout; cf. Taubes' quote from the review above). Those experts' judgements were based on review of studies on humans, non-experimental ('cohort' and 'case-control' studies) as well as experimental.

Based on its own reviews, the NCI places no "dietary factors" under "Risk factors causally associated with cancer" nor under "Risk factors with uncertain associations with cancer." It says only this:

Observational epidemiologic studies (case-control and cohort studies) have suggested associations between diet and cancer development, but randomized trials of interventions provided little or no support. ... Ecologic, cohort, and case-control studies found an association between fat and red meat intake and colon cancer risk, but a randomized controlled trial of low-fat diet in postmenopausal women showed no reduction in colon cancer. The low-fat diet did not affect all-cancer mortality, overall mortality, or cardiovascular disease.

Evidently, the NCI places more reliance on randomized trials than "ecologic, cohort, and case-control studies." But it leaves open the possibility that the trials have been about relatively short-term effects, which is not what the fat and carbohydrate hypotheses are about.

Apart from fats and carbohydrates in the macro-composition of diet, an eminent topic in respect to prevention/retardation of oncogenesis has been *micronutrients* in the diet, in a particular theoretical framework.

As Taubes explains, a normal feature of metabolism is "the production of ... *oxidants*, [which] *oxidize* other molecules ... The object of oxidation slowly deteriorates. ... *Antioxidants* neutralize [oxidants], which is why antioxidants have become a popular buzzword among nutritionists" (p. 191; italics in the original). Part of that deterioration occurs in the genome, as a matter of mutations possibly leading to turned-on oncogenes and turned-off tumor-supressor genes, which jointly constitute the deepest essence of cancer. Retardation of this genetic deterioration is the direct aim of recommending foods rich in antioxidants, and antioxidant supplementation of diet, in preventive oncology. The extent to which dietary antioxidants or their supplementations actually serve to slow down oncogenesis, or to delay/prevent overt cancer, Taubes does not discuss, as his interest focuses on the fact that increasing level of blood sugar – due to dietary carbohydrates – increases the production of those oxidants.

The WCRF/AICR report addresses mainly "*foods containing*" antioxidants – folate, carotenoids, beta-carotene, lycopene, vitamin C, selenium, pyridoxine, vitamin E, and quercetin. It associates the judgement of "convincing" or "probably" decreased risk of cancer with foods containing folate (oesophagus, pancreas, and colorectum), carotenoids (mouth, pharynx, larynx, and lung), beta-carotene (oesophagus), vitamin C (oesophagus), selenium (lung, stomach, colorectum, prostate), pyridoxine (oesophagus), vitamin E (oesophagus, prostate), and quercetin (lung). That is, it associates at least probable decrease in risk of some cancer or cancers with each of the foods containing antioxidants, except the dietary sources of lycopene.

In respect to antioxidant *supplementation* of diet this report addresses beta-carotene, selenium, retinol, and alpha-tocopherol. It associates convincing or probable increase (*sic*) of risk with beta-carotene (lung), neither convincing nor probable decrease of risk with retinol (any cancer), and either convincing or probable decrease of risk with selenium (prostate, lung, colorectal) and alpha-tocopherol (prostate).

The NCI site addresses "vitamin and dietary supplement use," under the rubric of "Interventions." The antioxidants among these have no representation at all under those "with proven benefits." Under the other rubric, those "with no proven benefits," the NCI paints the big picture thus:

> Some have advocated vitamin and mineral supplements for cancer prevention. Many different pathways for anticancer effects have been invoked. A commonly tested hypothesis is that antioxidant vitamins may protect against cancer, based on the premise that oxidative damage to DNA leads to cancer. However, the evidence is insufficient to support the use of multivitamin and mineral supplements or single vitamins or minerals to prevent cancer [ref.] ... Research into the potential anticancer properties of vitamin and mineral supplements is ongoing, and the results continue to reinforce the lack of efficacy of vitamin supplements in preventing cancer. Results from several large-scale randomized trials were published in 2009. [The supplementation] ... did not reduce ... had no benefit ... was not efficacious ... was not efficacious ... [produced] an increase ...

But again, were those randomized trials addressing the much-delayed effect of reduced DNA damage, in early life, on occurrence of overt cancer in middle age or later? See sections 7.1 and 7.2.

2.3 Nutrition and Ageing

'For reasons of symmetry,' as the saying goes, we could have invoked the neologism 'presbogenesis' à la 'atherogenesis' and 'oncogenesis' to denote the *process of biological ageing* (of tissues; Gr. *presbus*, 'old man').

From the vantage of nutrition and health, the ultimate concern is not the occurrence nor the nature of this process but the *rate* of it, its rate in causal relation to nutritional determinants of it, micronutrient supplementation of diet included. The slower is this rate, the longer tends to be (by a reasonable presumption) the *duration of life*, including life free of (overt) cardiovascular disease from atheromatosis and free of (overt, adult-onset) cancer. These 'degenerative' diseases (along with arthrosis and dementia, i.a.) can be viewed as largely being manifestations of relatively advanced stages of this (cumulative) presbogenesis.

Taubes (ref. in sect. 2.1) reviews "the spectacular benefits of semi-starvation on the health and longevity of laboratory animals" (p. 218 ff.). "The calorie-restricted animals live longer because of some metabolic or hormonal consequences of semi-starvation, not because they are necessarily leaner or lighter" (p. 219). And, back to his leit motif, he writes (pp. 219-20) this:

> The characteristics that all these long-lived organisms seem to share definitively are reduced insulin resistance, and abnormally low levels of blood sugar, insulin, and insulin-like growth factor. As a result, *the current thinking is that a lifelong reduction in blood sugar, insulin, and IGF bestows a longer and healthier life*. The reduction in blood sugar also leads to reduced oxidative stress ... [Italics ours.]

Remarkably, Taubes makes no reference to population-level epidemiological research on human nutrition and ageing, despite the great interest of people in this topic. It seems that this research has not yet really begun (cf. sect. 1.2). Alchemy, by contrast, represented a very determined long-term effort to develop an antidote to human ageing. As Jacob Bronowski explains in his *The Ascent of Man* (1972), alchemists' "search to make gold and to find the elixir of life are one and the same endeavor. … every medicine to fight old age contained gold … and the alchemists urged their patrons to drink from gold cups to prolong life" (p. 138).

2.4 Nutrition and Obesity

People's concern to preserve their health is most pronounced in such truly modern countries as the U.S.; and, as we've noted, this concern translates into preoccupation with diet first and foremost. In these countries, people's main dietary health-concern now most commonly is prevention and/or control of obesity.

Given the *major epidemic of obesity* that has emerged in the U.S. and elsewhere in the last few decades, public-health officials, too, now view obesity as the main diet-related health problem in countries such as the U.S. Their concern is accentuated by the common conception of obesity as a causal precursor of diabetes and cardiovascular disease.

In the context of this major epidemic there has been no commensurate surge in research into the etiology/etiogenesis of obesity – *barogenesis* could be the term for weight gain (Gr. *baros*, 'weight') – as the causation of weight gain has been taken to be obvious and well known, on a-priori grounds. Gary Taubes (ref. in sect. 2.1) addresses this situation quite critically.

Everyone concerned with this matter, Taubes included, is committed to the *first law of thermodynamics* – that of the conservation of energy – as it bears on the storage of energy (as fat) in adipose (fat) tissues: If over a given interval of time there is a given change in the amount of energy a person has stored as fat, this is associated with a corresponding, energy-equivalent cumulative difference, over that interval of time, between the person's energy intake (from diet) and energy expenditure (in physical activity, i.a.) – and conversely, of course.

The ordinary reading of this equivalence focuses on the idea – quite correct – that any induced imbalance/difference in the rates of energy intake and energy expenditure, cumulatively over an interval of time, produces its energy-equivalent change in the amount of adipose tissue. And from this flows, first, the idea that to avoid weight gain, the need is to see to it that the intake of energy does not exceed the expenditure of it, and, second, the idea that for weight reduction the need is to decrease the (weekly or so) *quantity* of one's energy intake and/or to increase that of energy expenditure (by increasing physical activity).

Taubes makes a strong case for believing, or at least seriously entertaining, an alternative idea: By suitably changing the *quality* of the intake of energy, the consequence is a metabolic change away from the propensity for excessive storage of energy in adipose tissues – even without any restriction in the quantity of the intake of energy. The qualitative change at issue is, again, *lesser consumption of carbohydrates*, refined ones and sugars in particular, naturally compensated for by greater consumption of fats and/or proteins (even *ad libitum*).

Taubes describes the extensive research in direct support of this idea, and how even the mechanism of the effect is understandable: Consumption of carbohydrates stimulates the pancreatic excretion of insulin, which promotes the entry of fatty acids – derived from carbohydrates in the liver – into adipose tissues; and insulin also inhibits their release from this storage.

As a matter of practicalities, sustained weight reduction by means of restricted intake of energy is generally unattainable because of inability to adhere to such a diet, while avoidance of carbohydrates can be maintained as a feature of lifestyle; and 'exercise' (physical activity) too is overadvertised: it increases (appetite and its consequent) energy intake in proportion to the energy expenditure (quite minor) in it. Taubes reviews the studies behind these understandings.

Taubes relates the appearance, in 1976, of Theodore Cooper, then U.S. Assistant Secretary of Health, as an expert witness before U.S. Senator George McGovern's committee which was developing its *Dietary Goals for the United States*. Cooper first testified that "the consumption of high carbohydrate sources with the induction of obesity constitutes a very serious public health problem in the underprivileged and economically disadvantaged" (p. 404).

But in response to the Senator's looking for a "rule of thumb," Cooper reversed that first statement: "I think in order to have an effective reduction in weight and a realignment of our composition we have to focus on fat intake" (p. 406). Taubes sees this as a turning point in both public policy and research on obesity:

"The shift in the nutritional wisdom was now taking place, driven by the contagious effect of Ancel Keys's dietary-fat/heart-disease hypothesis on the closely related field of obesity. Any diet that allowed liberal fat consumption was to be considered unhealthy" (p. 410). "The small contingent of influential nutritionists from Fred Stare's department at Harvard provide an example of how this process of entrenchment evolved. ..." (p. 411). "The result is an enormous enterprise dedicated in theory to determining the relationship between diet, obesity, and disease, while dedicated in practice to convincing everyone involved, and the lay public, most of all, that the answers are already known and always have been – an enterprise, in other words, that purports to be a science and yet functions like a religion" (pp. 451-2).

In closing here, an instructive vignette from earlier history. In his *Bismarck* (2011), Jonathan Steinberg describes one of that great statesman's sons, suffering from obesity, as having been helped to lose weight by following instructions from his doctor, Ernst Schweninger (p. 413). And then, with the Reich Chancellor himself, in 1883, again desperately sick, this son of his brought Schweninger to see him (p. 414) – also obese, and famously gluttonous to boot.

"Schweninger saved Bismarck's life by ... [prescribing] a new diet for the entire family – tea or milk with eggs for breakfast, a 'little' fish and roast meat (no vegetables) at noon, a small jug of milk at 4:00 and yet another in the evening"

(p. 416). "The pains, the facial neuralgia, and the headaches vanished. Bismarck was able to ride again. His weight began to go down, ... From 1886 on [till his death in 1898] he never went above 227 pounds, a perfectly reasonable weight for a man six feet four" (p. 415).

Bismarck retained Schweninger as his personal physician for the rest of his life, and "in gratitude Bismarck imposed his 'House Doctor' on the Berlin medical faculty, which regarded him as a charlatan and refused to talk with him" (p. 416).

2.5   Nutrition and 'Hypertension'

In public education about healthy diet, a very eminent recent governmental message in Canada has emphasized the need to change the typical *salt* (sodium chloride) consumption from the prevailing mean of over 8 g/day to less than 4 g/d for persons of all ages and with even lower target levels for those under 10 or over 50 years of age. In this aspect of diet the proximal concern is the level of blood pressure: prevention or amelioration of 'hypertension.' (This term is a common medical misnomer for relatively high blood pressure, which might better be termed *hemohyperbarism*; Gr. *haima*, 'blood,' Gr. *baros*, 'weight, pressure'). Hypertension, in turn, is of concern as a major cause of vascular disease (cardiac and cerebral).

Taubes (ref. in sect. 2.1) makes the point that "Systematic reviews of the evidence ... have inevitably concluded that significant reductions in salt consumption – cutting our salt intake in half, for instance, which is difficult to accomplish in the real world – will drop blood pressure by perhaps 4 to 5 mm Hg in hypertensives and 2 mm Hg in the rest of us. ... So cutting our salt intake in half ... makes [in proportional terms] little difference" (p. 146). Available not yet to Taubes but to the Sodium Working Group as background for its 2010 recommendations to Health Canada also was "A comprehensive review on salt and health and current experience of worldwide salt reduction programmes" by F.J. He and G.A. MacGregor, published in *Journal of Human Hypertension* 2009; 23: 363-84.

"Until the recent salt hypothesis began receiving serious attention in the 1960s," Taubes explains, "the investigators paid little attention to nutritional explanations for the rise in blood pressure that accompanied Western diets and lifestyles. ... Of course, the same societies that ate little or no salt ate little or no sugar or white flour, so the evidence supported *both* hypotheses, although the investigators were interested only in one" (p. 146).

"The laboratory evidence that carbohydrate-rich diets can cause the body to retain water and to raise blood pressure, just as salt consumption is supposed to do, dates back over a century. ... In the late 1950s, a new generation of investigators rediscovered the phenomenon, ... By the early 1970s, researchers had demonstrated that the water-retaining effect of carbohydrates was due to the insulin secreted, which in turn induced the kidneys to reabsorb sodium rather than excrete it, and that insulin levels were indeed higher, on average, in hypertensives than in normal individuals." (Pp. 148-9).

None of this accompanies the now-typical teaching about dietary sodium in Canada (or elsewhere). Similarly, the *adverse effects* of severely restricted intake of salt are left out of this health education.

2.6 *Epidemiologic Reviews* in Review

Epidemiologic Reviews, by its self-description, "is a yearly journal published by Oxford University Press ... for the Johns Hopkins Bloomberg School of Public Health and is sponsored by the Society of Epidemiologic Research and the International Epidemiological Association." It is a journal in the usual meaning that authors submit their articles to it. A sister publication of the *American Journal of Epidemiology*, it is "devoted to publishing comprehensive and critical reviews on specific themes once a year."

This journal thus is a source from which to learn, on superficial review of it already, what the topical concerns in the advancement of epidemiological knowledge in recent years have been, while the respective "comprehensive and critical reviews" reveal the corresponding states of the attained evidence and, one hopes, knowledge.

The yearly "specific themes" in the 2001–2011 period were these:

2001 – Prostate cancer
2002 – Clinical trials
2003 – Injury prevention and control
2004 – Social epidemiology
2005 – Epidemiologic approaches to disasters
2006 – Vaccines and public health
2007 – The obesity epidemic
2008 – The epidemiology of mental disorders
2009 – Epidemiologic approaches to health disparities
2010 – Epidemiologic approaches to global health
2011 – Screening

Some observations on select ones of these follow.

Given our fundamental tenet that epidemiology is (practice of) community medicine (sect. 1.1), we first examine the *2005 issue*, concerned with epidemiological approaches to *disasters*, to determine whether population-level medical care for disaster-afflicted populations was viewed as being epidemiology. Of main interest in this respect is the Editorial in that issue, by the eminent epidemiologist Michel Ibrahim.

"As evidenced in this issue," Ibrahim wrote, "epidemiology has an important role to play in the study of characteristics of populations affected by disasters and the deaths and injuries that follow. A seminal article ... shows epidemiologic approaches to disaster assessment at its best. ... As presented in several papers in this issue, epidemiologic methods and public health strategies are important in assessing and containing disasters. ... The time-honored prevention and control measures come into play: ... vaccinating high-risk groups against infectious diseases ... "

The final paragraph is particularly telling: "Now more than ever, public health preparedness has become a high priority of governments that must have the ability to predict, prevent, and control disasters and their consequences. Adequate funds are crucial to achieve this purpose, but epidemiologic know-how also has a role to play."

Now, as a disaster – an earthquake with or without a tsunami, say – produces public-health problems in terms of epidemics of injuries and other illnesses, it is, as Ibrahim said, the responsibility, specifically, of the governments' public-health officials "to predict, prevent, and control" these epidemics. The leading officials in this naturally are (practicing) epidemiologists. As remains commonplace, Ibrahim wrote about 'public-health' practices when at issue were, specifically, the epidemiological varieties of these (cf. sect. 1.1, i.a.). He wrote about epidemiologists in the practice of community medicine – in the practice of epidemiology, that is (cf. sect. 1.1).

Related to the essence of epidemiology, the point that *'social epidemiology'* now is on the ascendancy came up in section 1.4. And it is of note that in the period from 2001 to 2011, the *2004 issue* was expressly devoted to this, while related to this also was the 2009 issue. Suffice it here to quote from the Introduction to the 2004 issue, by Lisa Berkman:

> Social epidemiology, disguised in other forms and known by other names, has been with us for decades, if not centuries. ... the field is not a new one, nor are epidemiologists the only scientists contributing to a deepening understanding of the *social determinants of health*. ... I would argue that the important insights of social epidemiologists are based on the training they have in the assessment of health, disease, and biological pathways and the capacity to integrate 'upstream' social dynamics into their modeling of disease causation. [Italics ours.]

A fuller account of Berkman's – and others' – conception of social epidemiology can be found in *Social Epidemiology* (2000), of which Berkman and I. Kawachi are the Editors.

Of added note, a propos, eminently is *Epidemiology and the People's Health* (2011) by Nancy Krieger. She writes (p. 163) that,

> Among the extant social epidemiologic perspectives, I would argue three distinct theoretical trends exist. ... Of these, the first, *sociopolitical*, focuses principally on power, politics, economics, and rights as key societal determinants of health; the second, *psychosocial*, emphasizes psychosocially-mediated social determinants of population health. ... The third trend ... is more nascent and is best represented by *ecosocial theory*, which builds on and extends these first two frameworks by solving both the embodied population distributions of disease and health *and* epidemiologic theories of disease distribution, each in relation to their societal, ecological, and historical context. [Italics in the original.]

Given what 'social epidemiology' is said to be about, it is unsurprising that it is *not an outgrowth of epidemiology* in the research meaning of 'epidemiology.' It arose from *sociology*, and only quite recently (cf. Berkman above). As Krieger explains (p. 165),

By 1969, enough familiarity with the field exists that Leo G. Reeder presents a major address to the American Sociological Association called 'Social Epidemiology: An appraisal'
[ref.]. Defining *social epidemiology* as the 'study of the role of social factors in the etiology
of disease' [ref.], he asserts that 'social epidemiology ... seeks to expand the scope of
investigation to include variables and concepts drawn from a theory [ref.] – in effect, calling
for a marriage of sociological frameworks to epidemiologic inquiry. [Italics in the original.]

Recall, a propos, from section 1.4 a counsel of Francis Bacon: "Read not
to contradict, nor to believe, but to weigh and consider." Something to here
weigh and consider in particular is this: Given that epidemiological research
without the 'social' adjective addresses population occurrence of illness in relation
to characterizers of the population's individual members – their constitutional,
environmental, and behavioral characterizers – as a matter of *biomedical* research,
isn't it natural to think of study of the distribution of these determinants in
(human) populations/communities/societies as *social* and *behavioral* – rather than
biomedical – research, as a supplement to, rather than a type of, epidemiological
research? (Cf. sect. 1.4.)

And here is something more specific to weigh and consider. As epidemiologists
by their biomedical research have come to know how rates of various illnesses in
human populations are determined, causally, by the pattern of histories of, say,
smoking in the population, 'social epidemiologists' have nothing to add to this,
whatever may be their claims about "the training they have in the assessment
of health, disease, and biological pathways." By the same token, epidemiological
researchers of the established, biomedical variety are not experts on the patterns of
smoking in human populations and, especially, on how best to reduce these. They
defer to 'social epidemiologists' – a misnomer for *medical sociologists* – on this,
and, ultimately, to policy-promulgating societal authorities.

And finally here, while social epidemiology "has been with us for decades"
(Berkman, above), it remains inchoate: the order of the day evidently still is
conceptualization of what it is, rather than review of its accomplishments in the
advancement of the knowledge-base of community-level preventive medicine.

Epidemiological research and knowledge typically focus on a particular illness. It
thus is instructive to consider the *2001 issue*, focusing on *prostate cancer*. Following
a brief section on "descriptive epidemiology and natural history," most of that issue,
by far, was about factors in the causal origin – etiology/etiogenesis – of the illness:
"genetic factors," "hormones and growth factors," and "environmental factors" –
with diet classified as an environmental factor. There was, however, a short section
also on "prevention and control," addressing chemoprevention and screening.

A single article addressed "descriptive epidemiology," for which the term now is
'ecological epidemiology': "In this review," the authors said, "we present patterns
and trends of prostate cancer in various countries to provide further insights for
future epidemiologic studies." A propos, we remind the student that studies of
this type have had a major role in nutritional epidemiology (sects. 2.1, 2.2).
And we add that it has been commonplace to distinguish between 'descriptive'
and 'analytic' epidemiology, with the idea that studies of the former type serve

'hypothesis generation' (regarding etiogenesis), while hypothesis testing requires studies of the latter type, defined by the units of observation being individuals (rather than populations). Epidemiology in the research-discipline meaning of the term (sect. 1.3) focuses on 'analytic studies' (which term is as gross a misnomer in epidemiological research – its logic being synthetic – as its semi-cognate 'data analysis' – meaning data synthesis – is in statistics).

There was a single article on "natural history" of prostate cancer but it was not about the natural (untreated) course of the disease (for which the term is, in medicine, a commonly-used misnomer). Instead, surprisingly, "The intention of this brief review is to present some of the most pertinent facts regarding the pathobiology of prostate and its malignancies, and thereby facilitate the future work of epidemiologists studying this important disease." We very much agree with this intention: even if the conception of epidemiological research be limited to population-level occurrence research (sect. 1.2), knowledge about the anatomic site, pathology, and clinical aspects of the illness at issue may well "facilitate" the research; and it generally is essential for its scientific quality assurance.

A propos of section 2.2 above, it is of interest that one article did address fat intake in the etiogenesis of prostate cancer, and that none of them dealt with the etiogenetic role of the carbohydrate composition of diet. Illustrative of that particular review is this: "Data from several ecologic studies have shown positive correlations (r ≥ 0.6) between per capita intake of total, saturated, or animal fat and prostate cancer incidence or mortality [refs.]. ... Although several case-control studies found positive associations (odds ratio (OR) ≥ 1.3) between total fat intake and the risk of prostate cancer [refs.], only slightly fewer failed to find this relation [refs.]. ... Because cohort studies of diet and cancer avoid the problem of recall bias and are less prone than case-control studies to other [sic] selection biases, they are generally given more weight in overall assessments of the literature. Three such studies ... examined total fat and prostate cancer; two of these studies [refs.] found a positive association (relative risk ≥ 1. 3)."

So, with 'descriptive'/'ecologic' studies again the point of departure, the emphasis was on the now-perceived two principal types of 'analytic' study: 'case-control' and 'cohort' studies, the former producing findings in terms of 'odds ratio,' the latter in terms of 'relative risk' and both with no indication of what contrast (based on the quantitative determinant) was at issue. Review of the findings of a given one of the latter two types of study were taken to be a matter of noting what proportion of the studies "found a positive association" and what proportion "failed to find this relation." And the studies – none of them of 'basic' science – were seen to be marred by potential biases.

All of this is, at present, rather typical of epidemiological concepts, terminology, thinking, and writing; and we find it to be, in many ways, disagreeable. For a student these excerpts from this review are indicative of what now is out there, even if it remains far from being understood – correctly interpreted and evaluated. We present our critical understandings in the ensuing chapters, and we suggest that the student return to these passages for critical examination of them after having studied chapter 6 at least.

This review of dietary fat in the etiogenesis of prostate cancer was placed under the rubric of "environmental factors" as distinct from "genetic factors" and "hormones and growth factors," but we think in terms of a triad of categories for illness-causing factors: constitutional, environmental, and behavioral. All somatic factors, whether congenital (e.g., genetic) or 'acquired' (post-natally), we think of as *constitutional* (with "hormones and growth factors" among these). And we decisively separate *behavioral* factors – active ones of lifestyle, such as dietary habits – from factors that are, passively, *environmental* (from the vantage of a given person).

The last, brief section in this issue of the *Reviews* is noteworthy by its title: "Prevention and control." So, *prevention and control* of the occurrence of prostate cancer – these matters of practice – apparently were taken to be matters of epidemiology (rather than extra-epidemiological practice of public health). But this is not very clear from the three reviews under this rubric, one of them addressing chemoprevention of prostate cancer, the other two screening for it. However, one of the two screening reviews clearly went to matters beyond research, to matters of practice of screening:

> In summary, patients must be informed about the risks and benefits of prostate cancer screening before it is carried out. . . . If screening (and eventual treatment) is to be offered to asymptomatic patients, it should be offered to those in whom age and health status are such that they may benefit from early detection of a disease which may have a protracted natural history [meaning course in the absence of treatment; cf. above].

The current, major epidemic of *obesity*, in the U.S. and elsewhere (sect. 2.4), makes the *2007 issue* both timely and interesting.

The lead article, by B. Caballero, "provides an introduction to this issue" of the *Reviews*. It pointed out that,

> In spite of extensive research over the past decades, the mechanisms by which people attain excessive body weight and adiposity are still only partially understood . . . As discussed in this overview, there is an increasing consensus among obesity experts that changing the 'obesogenic' *environment* is a critical step toward reducing obesity. Reversing the factors . . . that lead to *increased caloric consumption* and *reduced physical activity* would require major changes in urban planning, transportation, public safety, and food production and marketing. [Italics ours.]

Caballero's overview is illustrative of the now-common thinking about diet as bearing on obesity through the *quantity* of its energy content, with no thought about the role of the *quality* of the diet in causing the metabolism to become "obesogenic" at whatever level (quantitative) of energy intake (cf. sect. 2.4). Curiously, diet and physical activity were here seen, à la "obesity experts," to be environmentally determined aspects of behavior.

Of the other articles in this issue of the *Reviews*, of particular note, a propos of the sections above, is that by R. Kelishadi: "In a systematic review . . . of the literature from 1950-2007, [he] compared data from surveys on the prevalence

of overweight, obesity, and the metabolic syndrome among children living in
developing countries. ... Time trends in childhood obesity and its metabolic
consequences ... should be monitored in developing countries in order to obtain
useful insights for primordial and primary prevention of the upcoming chronic
disease epidemic in such communities."

The definition of the *metabolic syndrome* in childhood and adolescence is
variable, an example of the definitions being that by Lambert et alii in a Canadian
study, as presented by Kelishadi: "Hyperinsulinemia combined with ≥ 2 risk factors
including overweight, high systolic blood pressure (>90th percentile), impaired
fasting blood glucose, high triglycerides (>75th percentile), and low HDL-c (<25th
percentile)." In this, non-metabolic elements are intermixed with metabolic ones.

Kelishadi made these remarks about actual risk factors of the metabolic syndrome:

> unhealthy dietary habits, particularly high carbohydrate and fat intakes, are associated
> with the metabolic syndrome in adults [ref.]. ... we found that the risk of the metabolic
> syndrome among children and adolescents rose with the consumption of solid hydrogenated
> fat and whole-flour bread [ref.]. While the frequency of intake of sweets (candies) increased
> the risk of the metabolic syndrome in both sexes, the frequency of eating fast foods and the
> frequency of eating carbohydrates increased the risk in boys and girls, respectively. In both
> sexes, the frequency of consumption of fruits and vegetables, as well as dairy products,
> decreased the risk of having the metabolic syndrome [ref.].

In this he repeatedly makes the common mistake of equating the finding of an
outcome-antecedent association with documentation of an effect-cause relation, as
though the latter were a phenomenon, subject to observation: X "increased the risk"
of Y ... See section 4.2.

In the Conclusion, very notably, there was nothing about dietary carbohydrates
in the etiogenesis of obesity and of its associated metabolic anomalies in the
metabolic syndrome. Instead, the review was said to have been about "childhood
overweight and its metabolic *consequences*" (italics ours). And as for the etiogenesis
of overweight/obesity, the conclusion was a simple affirmation of the prevailing
orthodoxy (sect. 2.4): "Strategies aimed at reducing caloric intake and increasing
caloric expenditure through regular exercise, early and aggressively, are necessary
..."

The *2011 issue* of the *Reviews*, on *screening* – a topic in respect to prostate cancer
already (above) – began with an Overview by R. Harris. Under the important
subheading of "Where we are and where we may be heading" he wrote this:

> Overall, then, the present truths about screening are that it is sometimes effective in
> improving health outcomes, that it is also associated with important harms, ... With few
> exceptions, the contribution of screening to improving the health of the public is small, ...
> Perhaps we should not think of screening as our primary prevention strategy but rather use
> screening to make a real, but limited contribution to population health for a few conditions.
> ... Fletcher's [ref.] thoughtful perspective on breast cancer screening is consistent with this
> vision of the future of screening. ...

S.W. Fletcher, whom Harris so put on a pedestal, wrote about "Breast cancer screening: A 35-year perspective." She made the familiar but ever-so-stunning points that "randomized trials of breast cancer screening have involved more than 650,000 women," and that "even so, no other cancer screening has produced such heated controversy. Multiple reviews have been published, . . ." See Appendix 2.

Regarding the formulation of ideas and recommendations about screening for a cancer, Fletcher described the pivotal roles that have been played by two "task forces," from the vantage of herself having been a founding member of both of them. She gave no justification for the formation, membership, or functioning of these task forces. See Apps. 1, 2, and 3.

"Both the Canadian and U.S. task forces emphasized the importance of *randomized trials* in their assessments of and recommendations for cancer screening" (italics ours). And illustrative of the results of these trials is this passage by Fletcher:

> The most recent meta-analysis [by the U.S. Preventive Medicine Task Force, of the results of the eight trials, having involved the total of over 650,000 participants, as noted above] found that breast cancer mortality reduction among women invited to screening was 15% for women aged 39-49 years, 14% for women aged 50-59 years, and 32% for women aged 60-69 years, with corresponding numbers needed to invite to screening to prevent 1 breast cancer death of 1,904, 1,339, and 377, respectively [ref.].

While presenting these numbers concerning mortality "reductions" that purportedly were "found" and purportedly implied – with four-digit accuracy! – various "numbers needed to invite to screening to prevent 1 breast cancer death" – irrespective of the nature and duration of the screening! – she had nothing to say about them, "thoughtful" or otherwise. See Appendix 2.

2.7 Overview of the Achievements

The aim of epidemiological research should be understood to be advancement of epidemiological practices in the improvement of population health in human communities. We defined epidemiological research by this aim of it, regardless of how 'basic' the research is (sect. 1.2). And we outlined the enormous achievements of epidemiological research, thus defined, in providing for the prevention and control of epidemics of communicable diseases (sect. 1.1).

Given that the accomplishments of epidemiological research and practice have been enormous in respect to communicable diseases and have more recently been extended to population-level prevention of illnesses of whatever kind (sect. 1.1), the question now is, specifically, about the accomplishments of the research in the advancement of the relatively novel types of epidemiological practice. We sought a partial answer to this question by focusing on *nutrition* as a determinant the health of populations (through its effects on individuals), health as for various diseases (incl. obesity) and longevity too (sects. 2.1, 2.2, 2.3, 2.4, 2.5); and we supplemented this by a cursory review of *Epidemiologic Reviews* (sect. 2.6).

The alert student will have taken note of the subtitle of Taubes' book (ref. in sect. 2.1), the element of *controversial science* in it. Taubes quotes Henry Blackburn, the eminent cardiovascular epidemiologist, as having written, in 1975, that "two strikingly polar attitudes persist on this subject [i.e., the etiology/etiogenesis of coronary heart disease, as to whether it has to do with fats or carbohydrates in the diet], with much talk from each and little listening between" (p. 22).

At the root of the controversies are, as Taubes explains, two aberrations of the culture surrounding epidemiological research: inattention to relevant 'basic' research and dogmatism, among the investigators and also the agencies sponsoring the research.

One of us was an author in a paper indicating that alcohol consumption indeed does prevent coronary heart disease. Puzzled why evidence of this had not been published from the Framingham Heart Study, in the 'blue books' of which the association (negative) had been quite apparent, he asked one of the FHS investigators about this. The answer was that this colleague himself actually wrote a manuscript on it. But: its approval process in the sponsoring agency – the National Heart and Lung Institute of the U.S. – went, quite exceptionally, all the way up to the head of the Institute; and he blocked the article's publication on the ground that knowledge of this salutary effect of alcohol consumption would promote alcoholism among the American people.

Taubes gives several examples of censorship, doctrinaire investigators' self-censorship as well as censorship by their sponsoring agencies. Particularly instructive about the role of institutional dogmatism are his descriptions of how institutional ideas – specifically of what the truth about the matter at issue is – play a role in the selection of like-minded experts to committees with the charge to review the evidence and to seek to determine what the truth is, thus making 'official' the conception of the truth that the agency already was holding.

In the framework of this culture surrounding the relevant scholarship, people have been taught, for decades, to avoid fats in their diets; and so they have consumed carbohydrates instead – and have grown obese, quite possibly as a consequence of this. Now, somewhat hesitantly, the reversal of this teaching is taking place; now the idea increasingly is that to be avoided are those carbohydrates, the consequence naturally being increase in the consumption of fats (and proteins too).

These matters should be seen to be at the very core of non-communicable, 'chronic' disease epidemiological research and knowledge. Yet the importance of them is not manifest in the topics addressed in *Epidemiologic Reviews* in 2001-2011. Moreover, these quite generally ignore the relevant 'basic' science and have no genuine knowledge to present. It took Taubes – a free-lance science-writer with no 'official' credentials in epidemiological research – to teach us about these matters, with unprecedented range of and depth of insights in the coverage.

To be sure, epidemiological research of this more recent, 'chronic-disease' genre (the dichotomy communicable vs. non-communicable actually is nowhere near coterminous with the acute-chronic dichotomy) has served to discover, and to an extent quantify, the effects of a large number of health hazards, those of cigarette *smoking* prime among these. But even in respect to this prime example, the history of progress is less than glorious: Franz Müller, in his medical thesis in Germany in 1939, gave quite compelling evidence to the effect that the main cause, by far, of the lung-cancer epidemic (which had been evolving for decades already) was smoking of cigarettes; and very strict anti-smoking policies were adopted in Germany, in part on the basis of this knowledge. Yet, as Robert Proctor in his *The Nazi War on Cancer* (1999) points out, "Wynder and Graham's famous paper from [1950] characterized tobacco merely as a 'possible etiologic factor' in the increase of the disease" (p. 196).

While Müller's study involved a mere 86 'cases' of death from lung cancer and 86 living and healthy 'controls,' 28 other 'case-control' studies with a total of 15,492 'cases' and 101,215 'controls,' and seven very large, expensive, and time-consuming 'cohort' studies – one of them with a cohort of 1,085,000 persons – were conducted before it got to be a piece of 'official' knowledge in the U.S. that smoking causes lung cancer. This landmark event took place as late as in 1964, in the form of the publication of the Surgeon General's *Smoking and Health* report. To say that which would go without saying, an enormous number of people have died of lung cancer as a consequence of their smoking in the quarter-century before 1964.

Given that epidemiological research has as its raison d'être the advancement of community medicine, there should be continual transmutation of epidemiological evidence into genuine epidemiological *knowledge*. The requisite innovations for the advancement of epidemiological knowledge we discuss in section 13.6 and in Appendix 3, while perfunctory programs to derive recommendations/guidelines for practice from evidence, without attention to expert knowledge, we address in Apps. 1 and 2.

While the *Epidemiologic Reviews* are supposed to be "comprehensive and critical," we find them to be strikingly uncritical – loose in both concepts and principles. The epitome of this lack of discipline (sect. 1.3) is the piece by an eminent 'clinical epidemiologist' – a founding member of the Canadian and U.S. task forces on "preventive" medicine – on an enormous amount of research that substantively has amounted only to "heated controversy," this on a topic that in critical conception is wholly extrinsic to preventive medicine! See Apps. 1 and 2.

Chapter 3
Etiology as a Pragmatic Concern

Abstract Epidemiological research is, almost exclusively, concerned with *etiology* of illness; but the concept of this remains quite generally misunderstood. To wit, according to *A Dictionary of Epidemiology* (2009) – a "handbook" sponsored by the International Epidemiological Association – etiology is "Literally, the science of causes, causality; in common usage, cause." (Tautology is not, literally or otherwise, the science of unnecessary repetition; nor is morphology, literally or otherwise, the science of shape, even though an important aspect of many sciences.)

For a student in an introductory course on epidemiological research it is essential to learn, for a start, that etiology – we prefer to term it *etiogenesis* (in analogy with 'pathogenesis' for the closely related descriptive concept) – is one of the two fundamental concepts of causation in medicine. And then the need is to learn, securely, the essence of this particular genre of causation in medical thought, to learn to distinguish it from *interventive* causality.

Once the medical concept of etiology/etiogenesis has been correctly introduced and internalized by the students, they are ready to be introduced to the role of etiogenetic knowledge in (the practice of) community medicine – in *community etiognosis*, preparatory to any action (education, regulation, or service) aimed at reduction of morbidity from some particular illness(es). In this etiognosis, general/abstract knowledge about etiogenesis is brought to bear on ad-hoc facts, to arrive at this particularistic type of knowing (about the causal origin of a given rate of morbidity in the community/population being cared for).

Community etiognosis (about a morbidity rate) has its counterpart in *clinical* medicine, focusing on a single case of an illness – or sickness not due to illness – and thus differing in its particulars from community etiognosis. The requisite knowledge is generally considerably more detailed/specific than in community etiognosis, and hence distinctly less secure (in today's context at least).

Clinical etiognosis is quite commonly a concern in *legal* contexts as well, but there it takes on a character different from what it is in clinical practice.

O.S. Miettinen and I. Karp, *Epidemiological Research: An Introduction*,   35
DOI 10.1007/978-94-007-4537-7_3, © Springer Science+Business Media Dordrecht 2012

3.1   The Two Genera of Causality in Medicine

Meteorological information merely *descriptive* of weather in a given place at a given time, present or prospective, is of value to the people in that place at that time. For, having such information people can make arrangements to adapt themselves to the weather; and even if this isn't their concern, they may appreciate the information out of sheer interest or curiosity. Of even greater, added value would be *causal* information about weather, were weather commonly to be subject to intentional change by human actions. In that case, information about existent weather would call for information also about meteorologic actions or inactions as causal explanations of it, and weather forecasts would be made conditional on what actions might, or will, be taken and would thus be made relevant for decisions about professional actions (prospective, communal) in the management of weather.

Like meteorological practice, medical practice too commonly is pursuit of certain facts and insights; but different from meteorology, medicine has been, for millennia already, much concerned with causality. In today's community medicine, the doctor – epidemiologist (sect. 1.1) – may proceed from community diagnosis – about the existent level of morbidity from a particular illness in the cared-for population – to consideration of the causal origin – etiology, *etiogenesis* – of this. And from morbidity diagnosis possibly supplemented by insight into the etiogenesis of the level of the morbidity – from community diagnosis possibly supplemented by community *etiognosis*, that is – (s)he proceeds to consider the future course of the morbidity, aiming to arrive at prognosis about this and, in particular, at *intervention-prognosis* to guide the decisions about the adoption of interventions. These two generic types of causality in community medicine – etiogenetic and interventive – have their obvious counterparts in clinical medicine, with presence/absence of a particular illness in place of the level of morbidity from it.

These two types of causal concern in medicine are very different, one from the other. Ad-hoc knowing about etiogenetic causality – etiognosis, that is (cf. above) – is tantamount to having a *causal explanation of an existent outcome* (level of a morbidity, or presence of an illness); it thus inherently is *retrospective* from the vantage of an existent outcome. By contrast, ad-hoc knowing about interventive causality is a decision-relevant input into prognosis; it is knowing about the *causal change in a future outcome* resulting from an intervention, the adoption of which (notionally or actually) is a given; it is *prospective* from the vantage of the decision about adoption (or continuation) of the intervention.

Despite this profound difference, these two types of causality in medicine share two important features. One of these is inherent in the very *concept of cause*. A potentially etiogenetic history, and a potentially outcome-changing intervention just the same, can be thought of as a potential cause only in the framework of a defined *causal contrast*: the potential cause being present (retrospectively or prospectively, according to which one of the two genera of causation is at issue) in lieu of its *defined alternative* being present. For example, thus, a given level of 'hypertension' (systemic) is a potential cause of the occurrence of stroke not per se but only if a lower level of blood pressure is taken to be the alternative (while with a higher BP the alternative, the given BP is a potential preventive – cause of non-occurrence – of stroke).

The other shared feature is this: Something that in general terms is a cause of the outcome need not be so in a particular instance, even when present; in a particular instance it is only a potential – possible – cause. Whether it in a given, individual instance actually was, or will be, causal will generally remain unknowable. On the individual, *clinical* level, only *probabilistic* knowing is realistic to pursue for etiognosis as well as for intervention-prognosis – *knowing about the probability* (objective) that the potential cause actually was, or will be, causal to the outcome's occurrence (its change from non-occurrence to actually occurring).

This said about the commonalities, another difference also is worth noting here. It has to do with the causal contrast, specifically with the causal determinant's *index category* in the contrast, representing the presence of the cause, as distinct from the reference category, representing the alternative to (rather than mere absence of) the cause. An etiognostic potential cause is *what it happens to be*: a particular pattern of the determinant status – constitutional, environmental, or behavioral – over the entire span of etiogenetically relevant time (retrospective), deviating from the corresponding, defined reference status throughout this period of time. In intervention-prognostic causation, by contrast, the potential cause is *what it is taken to be*, by choice, as for both its type and the duration of its implementation; it is algorithmic for the duration of its implementation (notional or actually planned), just as is its defined alternative.

Following these subtleties, it may be good to concentrate the mind by returning attention to the difference – profound – between the etiognostic and intervention-prognostic questions: In community medicine it is one thing to consider to what extent the current level of morbidity from a particular illness is due to the population's distribution by history in respect to a particular cause of it, this distribution's deviation from the reference distribution; and it is quite another thing to consider what would be the prospective change in that morbidity if a particular intervention were adopted (prospectively). The issue of the role of smoking in the etiogenesis of the prevailing rate of lung-cancer incidence is profoundly different from that of the change in this rate that would result from the adoption of a particular regulation concerning smoking, including as for the attainability of gnosis about it.

A modality of a doctor's action aimed at prevention of an illness in the client, in clinical as well as community medicine, commonly is *education* of the client (individual or population) about possible change in health-relevant lifestyle. This is not actual intervention on the course of the client's health, not intervention by the doctor nor by the client – any more than, say, 'intention-to-treat' based on randomization is actual intervention in an intervention trial. In community medicine, an actual intervention (preventive) is a change brought about by adopted public policy into the people's constitutions (as to, e.g., immunity), environments (e.g., pollution control), or behaviors (e.g., use of seatbelts). In clinical medicine an intervention is a physician-effected change in the client's constitution (e.g., by injection of a vaccine or a medication, or by tonsillectomy). Yet, even though prevention-oriented education of the client (population or individual) isn't actual intervention, it is justifiable – for simplicity and convenience – to subsume under 'intervention-prognostic' issues those that have to do with education about health-relevant aspects of lifestyle.

3.2   Etiology as a Community-medicine Concern

Apart from surveys and surveillances directed to health hazards and general promotion of healthy constitutions, environments, and behaviors in the cared-for population, a community doctor's concern is to get to know about the rates of morbidity from various illnesses in the population that (s)he is caring for – to achieve *community diagnosis* in this multifaceted sense – and then to devise specific ways of reducing those rates, 'unduly' high ones in particular.

Regarding a given one of those 'unduly' high rates, the epidemiologist's development of a plan to reduce it begins with his/her answer to the question, Why is this rate this high in this population at this time? What is causing this rate to be this high? The beginning of the control of morbidity from a particular illness thus is the answer – or the set of answers – to this question about etiology/etiogenesis, to this specifically *etiognostic question*. The rate at issue must be either specific in terms of its descriptive determinants or suitably adjusted for these, so that its high level does not have a descriptive, acausal explanation but needs a causal one.

Etiogenetic explanation of the rate of morbidity from a particular illness in a particular population at a particular time addresses the *proportion* of the rate that is caused by the factor at issue (by the pattern of its retrospective presence, in lieu of the defined alternative to this, in the members of the population). This is the proportion of the existing rate that would not be there but for the population's patterns of positive histories for the factor (*ceteris paribus*).

This explanation – the perception of this *overall etiogenetic proportion* – the epidemiologist can derive from two types of input. One of these types of input is, generally, peculiar to the cared-for population at the time in question. If the etiogenetic history is simply binary, such as use/non-use or seatbelt at the time of road accident, this first input is the proportion of the cases of the illness in which the affected person has the history of the factor/cause (non-use of seatbelt, say) having been present in the relevant past (i.e., in which the person had the index history and the case thus could have been caused by the factor at issue). This is the proportion of the cases of the illness – and hence of the rate of morbidity from the illness – that would be attributable to the factor were its presence (retrospective) always to be etiogenetic to cases of the illness occurring in association with its presence (retrospective).

The other input into the overall etiogenetic proportion – into the proportion now purportedly (ref. below) commonly termed 'attributable fraction (population)' – can be a matter of general epidemiological knowledge about cases of the illness that are associated with the potentially etiogenetic antecedent. It is the proportion of these antecedent-associated cases such that the antecedent actually is causal to the outcome, to the illness occurring – the *factor-conditional etiogenetic proportion* now purportedly (ref. below) properly termed 'attributable fraction (exposed).' The overall etiogenetic proportion for the cause at issue, in the population at the time, is the product of the two input proportions.

Reference: Porta M (Editor), Greenland S, Last JM (Associate Editors). *A Dictionary of Epidemiology*. A Handbook sponsored by the I.E.A. 5th edition. Oxford: Oxford University Press, 2008.

If the factor at issue is not of the all-or-none type but has, instead, more than a single index category, this calculation needs to be carried out separately for each of these. Then, the overall etiogenetic proportion is the sum of these component proportions.

Once the community doctor has a perception of the proportion caused by a given factor in the morbidity from a particular illness in the population (s)he is caring for, (s)he thereby has a sense – prognostic – of the extent to which that morbidity would be reduced if that factor were to be completely removed from the population; that is, if the prevailing distribution of histories concerning the risk factor at issue were to be replaced by their singularity representing the history's reference category. A regulatory intervention can have the potential to completely eliminate the cause-specific 'excess' morbidity from the illness at issue. But the adoption of a program of community-level health education, and the introduction of a prevention-oriented communal service just the same, when directed to a particular cause of morbidity, generally has a morbidity-reducing consequence that is an inestimable fraction of the etiogenetic proportion for the factor at issue. The inestimability of that fraction is mainly due to the unpredictability of the people's behavioral responses to the education about healthy lifestyles and of their actually making use of the preventive service(s) made available.

Any community-level health education directed to prevention would ideally be founded on knowledge that has evolved from etiognostic insights into expressly prognostic ones. The knowledge would ideally be specific to particular risk profiles of individuals in the population; and in reference to these it would address the way the prospective risk of the illness depends on the individual's prospective lifestyle in respect to the aspect of it that is at issue, or on the individual's use of preventive services – communal and/or clinical – so as to maintain particular levels of (patho)physiological risk factors for the illness. Presentation of this educational content would be complex, but it would be quite feasible via the Internet. The problem is the common unavailability, at present still, of such educational content. (Cf. ch. 2.)

3.3 Etiology as a Clinical-medicine Concern

When a clinician has arrived at a high-probability diagnosis (rule-in dgn.) about a particular illness, or strongly suspects a case of some sickness not to represent manifestation of any illness (somatic anomaly) but to be an adverse reaction to some exogenous agent (an ingested medication, say), (s)he is confronted with the clinical-type etiognostic question: Why is this person having this illness at this time? or, What agent is producing this adverse reaction in this person at this time? The former type of question (s)he may be able to regard as inconsequential, as the particular etiogenesis may not have implications for the management of the case at hand nor for prevention of recurrence of the illness. The answer to the latter kind of question, by contrast, is quite commonly consequential for the management of the case and practically always for prevention of its recurrence.

When setting out to meet this challenge, the clinician – in ideal practice at least – recalls the 'known' causes of the outcome at hand, ascertains the patient's history in respect to each of these, and translates these histories into the corresponding etiognostic probabilities. Relative to etiognosis about a particular cause in explaining a particular rate of morbidity in a practice of community medicine, the clinical situation is generally characterized by greater detail in the history about the potential cause and also about the 'host' of the outcome – about various aspects of the general etiogenetic triad (constitution/environment/behavior).

3.4   Etiology as a Legal Concern

In a court of law, the plaintiff in a 'class action' suit may be alleging that something industrial – a particular practice or environment or product – is causal to a particular illness experienced by people exposed to it; and in particular, that this is so in each case of the illness in a particular class of exposed people in general and, therefore, in each case among the members of the plaintiff 'class' of people. A case may also be brought to a court of law by an individual against a company or against his/her own doctor, alleging damage to his/her own health from an industrial environment or product or from a medical action.

The legal issue can be (as in the U.S.) whether the existence of the causal connection between the health outcome and its antecedent exposure is more probable than its non-existence. In a class action suit this has to do with such particulars of the exposure and the persons as are definitional to the class; and in the individual suit the issue is analogous to this, only more specific in its particulars.

In courts of law, just as in the practices of community and clinical medicine, there thus are issues about the etiology/etiogenesis of illness. But arguably different from medical practices, the legal practices related to etiogenesis of illness should involve express focus on the general question of *what is known* – in the community of the relevant experts – about the causal connection at issue, about the *probability* of its existence in such individual cases as the one(s) at issue. The relevant knowledge is about the *proportion* of instances like the one(s) at issue in general such that the antecedent is causal to the outcome, this proportion being the probability in question. Given the amount of relevant detail on an individual plaintiff, the knowledge-base for rational resolution of the legal cases tends not to derive satisfactorily from epidemiological (population-oriented) research on etiogenesis; it tends to require *clinical* (individuals-oriented) research of this genre.

Judges and lawyers cannot be presumed to understand the causality issues in these cases, notably as to the state of the scientific knowledge; they should be deferential to *experts* on the topic in question. They need to appreciate that science can, in principle at least, address such topics as the probability that a given medication use was causal to a particular adverse health event that has occurred in association with it, even though there can be no science to address the probability that a given person was causal to – guilty of – a tort or crime that has occurred.

This deference involves, in the context of the present state of science-based epidemiological – and meta-epidemiological clinical – knowledge (sect. 2.6), the problem that 'experts' are likely to have only widely-divergent personal opinions about the level of the probability in question, in lieu of actual knowledge about it.

So, in matters of science, even, the courts actually are down to witness testimonies separately for and against the causality in the case(s) at issue, generally by pseudo-experts. The only difference is that these witnesses present opinions about the probability regarding which the decisive opinion still is that of the judge or the jury – instead of merely presenting evidence relevant to that ultimately-relevant opinion.

Chapter 4
Etiology as the Object of Study

Abstract Research on etiogenesis of morbidity – or of illness per se – is, by the very nature of this genre of causation in medicine, generally bound to be *non-experimental*; but a much greater added challenge is that causation is not a phenomenon, subject to observation; it is a 'conception a priori,' a *noumenon* (Kant), needing to be inferred from phenomenal patterns.

If etiogenesis were a phenomenon, study of it would be based on a mere *case series* of the illness, the cases selected independently of their etiogenetic backgrounds, and the concern in it would be the proportion of the cases with the antecedent at issue such that the antecedent actually was (seen to be) causal to the case – this *factor-conditional etiogenetic proportion*.

But as etiogenesis is but an unobservable noumenon, the inescapably needed case series is to be an element in documentation of a phenomenon: the cases' rate of occurrence in a defined *study base*, the necessary added element being a sample of that study base, a *base series* that is.

The case and base series, considered jointly, allow for documentation of the relative levels of the rates of the cases' occurrence in segments of the study base, and of interest here are the rates for the index and reference segments of the study base – the rates for those with a positive history for the etiogenetic factor and for its alternative, respectively. The *rate ratio* for this contrast allows for calculation of a first approximation to the factor-conditional etiogenetic proportion (cf. above).

When, as is usual, the index and reference segments of the study base have different distributions by extraneous determinants of the cases' occurrence, control of this *confounding* is needed.

One option in this control is suitable '*standardization*' of the rate ratio. But this intuitively appealing approach is impracticable when the number of confounders is appreciable.

This limitation of the standardization approach to the control of confounding is avoided by invocation of a suitable *model* for the cases' rate of occurrence. A suitable log-linear model implies the rate ratio as a function of its modifiers,

O.S. Miettinen and I. Karp, *Epidemiological Research: An Introduction*,
DOI 10.1007/978-94-007-4537-7_4, © Springer Science+Business Media Dordrecht 2012

conditionally on the set of confounders and thus, free of confounding by them, and calculation of this result for the factor-conditional etiogenetic proportion can be based on this function's fitted counterpart.

4.1 Some Introductory Examples

1. Policies about DUI. Legal and other public-policy stipulations about DUI (driving under the influence, of alcohol) are principally guided by information about the 'excess' rate of fatal injuries that in the population within the policy-makers' purview is attributable (causally) to people's DUI, as defined, perhaps distinguishing among some demographic strata (by categories of age, most notably).

This DUI-attributable 'excess' rate of car-accident fatalities (in a given demographic stratum, say) is the overall rate of these fatalities in the population in question, regardless of causation, multiplied by the proportion of the overall rate that is attributable to DUI; and the latter, that overall etiologic/etiogenetic proportion, in turn, is the product of two proportions: the proportion – particularistic, in the population at the time – of the fatalities occurring in association with DUI, and the proportion – more-or-less general – of DUI-associated fatalities that actually are DUI-attributable (sect. 3.2). The latter proportion presumably is practically invariant over whatever demographic strata of the population of public-policy concern (so long as the distribution of the severity of the inebriation is practically the same over the strata).

It thus is knowledge of the *etiognostic*, rather than intervention-prognostic, type – from etiologic/etiogenetic research – that matters in this example; and that other type of research-based knowledge wouldn't even be practical to pursue for the purpose here (see below).

2. Policies about seatbelt use. The requisite knowledge-base for public policies about seatbelt use is, in its nature and genesis, quite analogous to that concerning DUI; but the other genre of causal research is now realistic – and instructive – to consider.

In the spirit of intervention-prognostic research (sect. 3.1), one would think of, and address, drivers staying in a given category of the risk factor (use/non-use of seatbelt) over considerable amounts of accrued mileage; and the study would address the incidence of fatal injury to the driver, from traffic accidents, for the contrasted categories. For categories of appreciable degrees of inebriation the capturing of this type of experience is quite unimaginable, but for driving with and without the use of the seatbelt it isn't.

Even though rather practicable in respect to seatbelt use, that alternative to the etiognostic outlook and approach is not the preferable one in this case, either. The rate has a multitude of determinants, both causal and acausal, other than the use/non-use of seatbelt. In the face of this complexity, sufficient for policies about the use of seatbelt is knowing its consequent proportional reduction – general – in the rate, this reduction in conjunction with what the rate – local – in the absence of seatbelt use is or would be. The relevant absolute reduction in the rate is the product of these two (cf. sect. 3.2), that general input into it naturally taken to be independent of that ad-hoc input.

So, again, the *etiognostic* genus of causal research is sufficient – while also obviously simpler than its intervention-prognostic alternative.

3. Policies about smoking. Like DUI and non-use of seatbelt, smoking is a matter of people's *behavior* that is of concern to promulgators of societal policies directed to promotion and preservation of public health (i.e., the health of the population in the policy-makers' purview; sect. 1.1). But the legal-regulatory stipulations restricting the people's admissible behaviors are in this context supplemented by regulation of the people's *environments:* the concern is not only to ban smoking in various particular types of setting; the people's environments are controlled as to whether, or what types of, tobacco products can be available (where and to whom, according to age). Another difference is that community-level health *education* about the behaviors – their health implications – is promoted by the policies – being that the risky behavior in many settings remains admissible (different from the examples above).

The policy-makers' direct concern is to reduce *morbidity* from illnesses for which smoking is etiogenetic, especially from illnesses through which smoking is a material contributor to *mortality* in the population. They thus need to learn – from the epidemiologist(s) caring for the population – in respect to illnesses such as lung cancer the prevailing rate of mortality in the population; or, more to the point, they need to learn the total mortality from smoking-related illnesses in the aggregate. And they need to learn the proportion of this mortality – really of the underlying morbidity – that is attributable (etiogenetically) to the people's (histories of) smoking (sect. 3.2).

In these, essential terms the scientific knowledge-base of public policy about smoking is analogous to that of the two examples above, with the relevant knowledge from epidemiological research again being of the *etiognostic* rather than of the intervention-prognostic type. A difference is, however, that smoking as the etiogenetic factor does not explain (causally) a proportion of the cases that is anywhere near invariant across all demographic strata of the population of concern. Regarding age in particular, the general (epidemiological) knowledge needs to be stratum-specific, including in respect to the typical positive history of smoking in materially relevant respects.

Once thus informed about the 'excess' mortality from smoking-related illness (by categories of age, at least), the regulators would like to have an added input into their decisions about the various possible regulatory interventions under consideration, namely the *intervention-prognostic* magnitudes of the effects of these (also by categories of age, at least). Knowledge about the magnitudes of these effects is, however, very impractical to acquire by epidemiological (or other) research. But it also is rather immaterial for the regulatory decisions, as cost-effectiveness is not really an issue in these decisions.

For community-level health *education* about smoking-related life-styles, it is essential to have research-based knowledge – sketchy knowledge at least – about the health – notably survival – implications of the principal choices that individuals in the population may make for themselves. These are the choices of whether to take up smoking and, insofar as one has taken it up, whether to quit the habit. For the development of this knowledge-base for health education, etiognostic research is both relevant and feasible, while prognostic research is quite problematic on account of the instability of the smoking habit among those who ever take up the habit – including incompleteness of the follow-through with decisions to permanently quit smoking.

4. Policies about fluoridation of drinking water. When behavioral etiogenetic factors such as DUI or non-use of seatbelt or smoking are removed from a population, this scarcely has adverse consequences on public health in terms of increase in morbidity from some illness(es) to which the behavior change was not directed. The same quite obviously is true of removing some pathogenetic agent from people's environments – airborne asbestos, for example.

Matters are different in respect to *micronutrients*, whether in food or drink or taken in as dietary supplements. Whereas all types of tissue in the human body have the same, known optimum (i.e., zero) for the concentration of the ingredients of tobacco smoke, for instance, this may not be the case for a given micronutrient. Fluorine appears to be a case in point.

Fluorine intake is essential for the health of bones in particular, freedom from dental caries included; and while the sources of this micronutrient include sea fish and tea, among others, the principal source generally is drinking water.

Etiogenetic research has produced the understanding that fluorine concentration less than 1 ppm in drinking water is causal to dental caries (while high concentrations, such as 10 ppm, cause pathologic fluorosis of bones, including teeth); and this understanding has led to policies of fluoridation of the drinking water in various municipalities with naturally low concentrations of fluorine. Predictably, this has had the consequence of reduced rates of dental caries in those municipalities.

But, no biological principle is to the effect that a level of fluorine intake that is optimal for dental health also is optimal for all other aspects of health – for minimizing the rate of oxidative genetic damage and of its resultant development of oncogenes and then cancers, for example. Concerns about adverse side effects of fluoridation of drinking water as for morbidity from illnesses other than dental caries have indeed arisen, and some programs of such environmental adjustments have been discontinued on this basis.

Intervention-prognostic studies on this topic, with attention to all outcomes potentially affected, would have provided the knowledge-base for these interventions, had they been practicable in the face of the need for a large number of municipalities and a very long-term follow-up (in respect to potential carcinogenesis in particular). But as they haven't been and perhaps won't be, etiogenetic studies based on naturally varying levels of fluorine in drinking water need to be extended to health outcomes other than dental caries.

4.2   From Case Series to Rate Comparison

Very important to appreciate about causation is the fact that it is not a phenomenon, that it thus is not subject to being observed. It is, instead, what Immanuel Kant termed a conception a priori, a *noumenon*. In this sense, as Kant points out, causation is akin to, say, space and time – not formed by experience but innate.

The concept of causation, noumenal as it is, has been remarkably baffling to many notable philosophers. Insofar as the Greek *aitia* (etymologic to the etio- prefix) can justifiably be translated as 'cause,' Aristotle envisioned four fundamental genera of cause: material, formal, effective, and final; but of these, only 'effective' aitia actually is a cause – and specifically etiogenetic/etiognostic rather than intervention-prognostic cause (sect. 3.1) – in our contemporary meaning of 'cause.'

William of Ockham (1285?–1349?) is now commonly (though falsely) taken to have been the originator of the important *principle of parsimony* (*L. parsimonia*, 'frugality'), namely that concepts are not to be multiplied beyond necessity; and one of his applications of this principle was advocacy (sharp, as usual, à la 'Ockham's razor') of seeing causation to be an unnecessary concept, an undeserving supplement to that of 'regular succession.' Similarly, the eminent empiricist philosopher David Hume (1711–1776) argued that knowable only is 'constant conjunction,' in lieu of causation. And subsequent 'positivist' philosophers, even of the twentieth century, had no use for noumenal concepts, such as causation.

Philosophers, while much concerned to understand what is and what is not 'real' (ontologically admissible to consider), have thus been conspicuously out of touch with the realities of medicine. Hippocrates (460? BCE–370? BCE), already, is taken to have brought forth the fundamental idea that illnesses are not divinely instigated; that instead, the beginning of the disease process is an offending material (*materia peccans*) bringing the bodily humors (blood, phlegm, yellow bile, and black bile) into a state of bad mixture (*dyskrasia*). Akin to this, a subsequent concern in medicine has always been to understand the occurrence of an illness (individually or in a population) as a matter of *causal explanation*, and beyond this, to *intentionally cause a change* in a person's or population's health for the better (cf. sect. 3.1). Without the concept of causation medicine would be as passive about people's health as, say, philosophers commonly elect to be about everything in their surrounding reality (insofar as they, perhaps only grudgingly, grant its existence) and cosmologists necessarily are about the goings-on in the cosmos.

In this aloofness from reality, philosophers have been in the Platonic mode. "To his persona as the first academic [Plato] added or superimposed the complementary persona of the first intellectual, by which I mean someone who thinks ideas matter more than people." So writes the eminent historiographer Paul Johnson in his *Socrates: A Man of Our Times* (2011; p. 11).

To gain the most fundamentally orientational understanding of what an etiologic/etiogenetic study is to be empirically about, it is helpful to first consider the thinking that would be natural *if causation were a phenomenon*. In this situation (counterfactual; cf. above) causation would be observable (and documentable) in each instance in which an antecedent (identifiable) actually is causal to a subsequent (also identifiable), serving to produce (*sic*) the subsequent – this outcome – while its defined alternative would not have had this effect (cf. sect. 3.1).

In this hypothetical situation, any etiogenetic study would focus on *cases of the illness*; and among these the narrower focus would be on the ones *associated with the antecedent* in question, as non-causation in the absence of the potential cause at issue is obvious a priori. In respect to these illness-antecedent instances, the object of study would be *the proportion of them such that the antecedent is causal –* etiogenetic – to the illness. The magnitude of this proportion would be directly studyable on the present premise – as a function of determinants of its magnitude – on the basis of its empirical counterpart in a case series of the illness.

An added object of study (scientific) would commonly be the proportion of the cases that are associated with the antecedent in question, if this commonly were a parameter – constant – of Nature. But it actually is prone to be an ad-hoc matter, devoid of universality (cf. sect. 4.1). Scientific study of this proportion, when meaningful on account of its universality, is not made more challenging by the fact that causation is a noumenon rather than a phenomenon.

Implicitly, in these remarks, at issue has been a (potential) cause of the all-or-none type, one without subtypes (by intensity or duration, say) to be distinguished. Insofar as there are such subtypes, those remarks apply to each of these separately, to each index category vis-à-vis the shared reference category.

In the real world the need is to move away from consideration of that un-observable etiogenetic proportion for a given index history in a series of cases of the illness with the antecedent, to consideration of certain related, inherently observable, *phenomena*: that proportion's manifestation in *rates* into which the case series supplies numerator inputs. To this end it is necessary to think of the case series as constituting those occurring in a defined experience of the cases' potential occurrence, the experience – the *study base* – classified according to whether the antecedent in question was present, or the alternative to this was, or neither one of these was.

Focusing on the empirical rates R_i and R_0 for the respective experiences with the *i*th index category of the antecedent and the reference category (present retrospectively as of the outcome; sect. 3.1), the *factor-conditional etiogenetic proportion* addressed above is, to a first approximation,

$$(R_i - R_0)/R_i = (RR_i - 1)/RR_i,$$

where $RR_i = R_i/R_0$, the *i*th rate ratio, the *index rate* divided by the *reference rate*.

This measure of the etiogenetic proportion of interest, while based on phenomena (rates), adduces a new challenge: the magnitude of this RR_i, based on 'crude' (unadjusted) overall rates as it is, can have *extraneous explanations* in addition to the etiogenetic proportion in question; therefore, the need is to consider the corresponding RR_i that is not subject to extraneous explanation.

4.3   Standardized RR as the Result

When epidemiologists in their practice of community medicine (sect. 1.1) compare two or more rates, there commonly is a need to 'adjust' one or more of the directly available, 'crude' overall rates for the compared experiences to achieve 'comparability' – most commonly so as to eliminate the role of the differential distributions of the respective populations by gender and age. The common means of this adjustment is mutual 'standardization' of the compared rates.

Following this practice as the paradigm leads to replacement of a 'crude' comparative measure, the crude RR_i in section 4.2 above, by the corresponding *standardized RR$_i$*, involving mutually standardized rates in lieu of the corresponding crude ones. The magnitude of a suitably standardized RR cannot be explained, even in part, by the difference in the compared populations' distributions by the determinants of the rate that were standardized for. In this way, *confounding* by differential distributions of the compared experiences according to those extraneous determinants of the outcome's rate of occurrence is 'controlled' – excluded from being a possible explanation of the magnitude of the result, the empirical comparative measure, that RR_i, notably its deviation from the null value of $RR_i = 1$.

The principle underlying this standardization of empirical rates is founded on the *latent structure of any crude overall rate*. With C the total number of cases of an illness occurring in PT amount of population-time, the crude overall rate, C/PT, is a (latently) 'weighted' average of the 'specific' rates in the 'strata' (by gender and age, say, here indexed by $j = 1, 2, \ldots$) contributing to the crude overall rate:

$$C/PT = \sum_j C_j / \sum_j PT_j$$

$$= \sum_j PT_j \left(C_j/PT_j\right) / \sum_j PT_j$$

$$= \sum_j PT_j R_j / \sum_j PT_j$$

$$= \sum_j \left(PT_j/PT\right) R_j / \sum_j \left(PT_j/PT\right)$$

$$= \sum_j W_j R_j,$$

where $\sum_j$ denotes summation over the strata ($j = 1, 2, \ldots$) and $W_j = PT_j/PT$ is the *latent weight* for the *specific rate*, $R_j = C_j/PT_j$, in the jth stratum. ($\sum_j W_j = 1$).

Given this structure of a crude rate, it follows that two or more rates are mutually *standardized* for one or more stratification factors if they involve the same ('standard') set of weights for their stratum-specific component rates. And a *standardized rate ratio* is based on two mutually standardized rates.

The implication of this standardization principle here is this: Of the crude index rate, R_{1i}, among those with the ith index history for the potentially etiogenetic factor in the study base, the proportion actually caused by the factor – the factor-conditional etiogenetic proportion (sect. 3.2) – is addressed by

$$\left(\widehat{RR}_i^* - 1\right)/\widehat{RR}_i^*,$$

where $\widehat{RR}_i^*$ is the standardized rate-ratio in a particular meaning. First, $\widehat{RR}_i^*$ involves R_{1i}, the crude – unadjusted – index rate (conditional on the ith index history). Second, it involves R_{0i}^*, the reference rate adjusted to the latent structure of the index rate (of its denominator input). And third, this adjustment of R_{0i} involves *all* extraneous determinants (acausal as well as causal) of the reference rate in terms of which the index and reference experiences differ.

While any choice of shared weights generally serves the purpose of standardization (attainment of comparability in particular respects), here the *weights* need to be thought of as those that are latent in the crude *index* rate (which rate therefore needs no adjustment for the $\widehat{RR}_i^*$). For only with these weights does the $\widehat{RR}_i^*$ represent the empirical value of the factor-conditional etiogenetic proportion – the proportion of the cases with the antecedent that are caused by the antecedent (sect. 3.2).

It is good to learn to think about this $\widehat{RR}_i^*$ as the '*observed-to-expected*,' or O_i/E_i, ratio of the number of cases in the index experience of the study base:

$$\widehat{RR}_i^* = (C_i/PT_i)/\left[\sum_j (PT_{ij})\, R_{0j}/\sum_j PT_{ij}\right]$$

$$= (O_i/PT_i)/\left(E_i/\sum_j (PT_{ij})\right)$$

$$= O_i/E_i.$$

Actually, this E_i is only the empirical counterpart of the actual null value corresponding to O_i, and we hence prefer the notation in

$$\widehat{RR}_i^* = O_i/\hat{E}_i.$$

While this standardization-based principle is impeccable in its logic, it adduces *two problems* to consider. For one, as noted above, it implies the necessity – inescapable need, throughout non-experimental etiogenetic research – to know what all of the extraneous determinants of the magnitude of reference rate are. And for another, given this knowledge – merely presumptive – standardization-based isolation of the purely causal RR_i^* is prone to be impracticable in the context of the generally large number of potential confounders.

For the latter problem there commonly is, in principle, a reasonable solution: the invocation of a suitable *model*.

4.4 The Object Imbedded in a Model

As background, or the context, for etiologic/etiogenetic modeling, let us recall the relevant essentials from section 4.3 above in reference to an antecedent of the all-or-none type:

1. An etiogenetic study has to do with instances – in a defined abstract domain – of the illness occurring in association with the antecedent whose etiogenetic role is at issue; and in elementary terms, the natural object of study is the proportion of these instances, in that domain, such that the antecedent actually is causal to the outcome.

2. The empirical value for this (factor-conditional etiogenetic) proportion (P) derives from the proportional extent to which a certain rate (R_1) exceeds another rate (R_0^*):

$$\hat{P} = (R_1 - R_0^*)/R_1$$
$$= (R_1/R_0^* - 1)/(R_1/R_0^*)$$
$$= (\widehat{RR}^* - 1)/\widehat{RR}^*$$
$$= (O/\hat{E} - 1)/(O/\hat{E}),$$

where R_1 is the crude index rate (with positive history for the factor at issue) and R_0^* is the reference rate (with positive history for that factor's defined alternative) adjusted to the latent structure of R_1 in respect to all extraneous determinants (acausal as well as causal) of the reference rate in terms of which the latent structures of the crude index and reference rates (R_1 and R_0) differ, these rates characterizing an experience in the domain of the object of study; and where O is the 'observed' number of cases contributing to the index rate and $\hat{E}$ is the corresponding null-expected number's empirical counterpart.

This is the standardization approach to obtaining an empirical value for the core object of an etiogenetic study – the study result in terms of the $O/\hat{E}$ ratio – serving to derive the corresponding result for the factor-conditional etiogenetic proportion. Involved is maintenance of the occurrence relation's conditionality on extraneous determinants of the outcome's rate of occurrence – of the reference rate, that is.

This leads to consideration of the outcome's rate of occurrence as a *joint function* (descriptive) of the etiogenetic determinant at issue and the presumedly inclusive set of the reference rate's extraneous determinants involved in the needed conditionality. In the framework of such a joint function the relation of the rate to the determinant at issue is inherently conditional on the set of extraneous determinants, given that the form of the function is realistic.

In an extremely simple situation the etiogenetic determinant would have only three (nominal) categories – index, reference, other – and the conditioning would involve only, say, gender and age. The correspondingly designed function – the *occurrence relation* designed as the *model* for the rate, R – might be as simple as

$$R = B_0 + B_1X_1 + B_2X_2 + B_3X_3 + B_4X_4,$$

where the *B*s are (presumed) *parameters* (constants) of Nature and the Xs are (ad-hoc adopted) *statistical variates* (which the determinants they represent aren't):

X_1 = indicator of index history (X_1 = 1 if this, 0 otherwise)
X_2 = indicator of 'other' history (so that $X_1 = X_2 = 0$ implies reference history)
X_3 = indicator of male gender
X_4 = age as the number of years (i.e., age/yr).

What is simple about that situation is not merely the all-or-none nature of the set of possible etiogenetic histories and the (presumed) need to condition the relation of R to these on gender and age only; and an added simplicity is the feature that R is a numerical quantity – not incidence density but a proportion-type rate (of incidence or prevalence).

And for that simple situation that model is quantitatively simple in two of its implications: that the magnitude of the effect at issue (the difference between R_1, involving $X_1 = 1$ together with $X_2 = 0$, and R_0, involving $X_1 = X_2 = 0$) is constant (B_1) over (i.e., unmodified by) gender and age; and that full conditioning by gender and age is provided for by their very simple – simply additive – representation in that model (without, say, $X_5 = X_4^2$, $X_6 = X_3X_4$, and $X_7 = X_3X_5$).

In terms of the fitted counterpart of this simple model we have $\hat{R}_{0j}$ defined for each of the strata by gender and age (focusing on typical age in each stratum). The standardized reference rate R_0^* corresponding to the crude index rate R_1 is $\sum_j W_j\hat{R}_{0j}$, where the weights derive from the index experience. Then, $R_1/R_0^* = O/\hat{E}$ implies the empirical value for the factor-conditional etiogenetic proportion (see above).

The stratification in the derivation of the $O/\hat{E}$ ratio actually is unnecessary. Associated with each index case (among the O number of these) is the corresponding $\hat{R}_{1j}$ and $\hat{R}_{0j}$ implied by the fitted model; and hence the corresponding $\widehat{RR}_j$ also. Thus,

$$\hat{E} = \sum_j 1/\widehat{RR}_j,$$

where the summation is over the index cases (O in number), their profiles in terms of gender and (actual) age.

A slightly but importantly modified version of that simple model is this '*log-linear*' one:

$$\log(R) = \sum_0^4 B_iX_i,$$

where $X_0 = 1$. The modification is that the 'linear compound' (of the Bs, with the Xs the 'coefficients' in it) now represents the magnitude of the logarithm (natural, Napierian) of the numerical (dimensionless) rate. In terms of this model,

$$\log (R_1) - \log (R_0) = B_1$$
$$\log (R_1/R_0) = B_1$$
$$R_1/R_0 = \exp (B_1),$$

where 'exp' denotes 'exponential of'; that is, 'antilog (base e) of.'

Insofar as this model is correct – as to its implication that the difference in $\log (R)$ corresponding to $X_1 = 1$ (and $X_2 = 0$) versus $X_1 = 0$ (and $X_2 = 0$) is constant over gender and age, and the bearing of gender and age on $\log(R)$ is correctly represented in reference to the subdomain in which $X_1 = 0$ (and $X_2 = 0$) – the implication is that the model's fitted counterpart implies

$$\widehat{RR}^* = O/\hat{E} = \exp (B_1).$$

If, however, the model should additionally include

$$X_5 = X_1 X_3,$$

the implication would be that

$$\log (R_1) - \log (R_0) = B_1 + B_5 X_3,$$

implying gender modification of the RR:

$$RR = \exp (B_1 + B_5 X_3)$$
$$= \exp (B_1) \text{ given } X_3 = 0 \text{ (female gender)}$$
$$= \exp (B_1 + B_5) \text{ given } X_3 = 1 \text{ (male gender)}.$$

This model thus implies directly the gender-specific values of the RR but the overall RR^* only through the values of R_{1j} and R_{0j} it thus defines (cf. above).

But, as noted above, this stratification actually is unnecessary. Log-linear models for a rate, whether a proportion-type rate per se or the numerical element in incidence density, are the ones of principal concern in etiogenetic research. Without having to derive values of $\hat{R}_{1j}$ and $\hat{R}_{0j}$, the values of $\widehat{RR}_j$ are obtained directly from the fitted RR function (of its modifiers). Then, as above,

$$\widehat{RR}^* = O/\hat{E} = C_1 / \sum_j \left(1/\widehat{RR}_j \right),$$

where C_1 is the number of index cases of the illness (ones occurring in association with the antecedent at issue), the summation is over all of these cases, and $\widehat{RR}_j$ is the empirical RR corresponding to the modifier profile of the jth one of these cases.

This point likely deserves to be restated, though somewhat differently. Log-linear modeling of the rate at issue in etiogenetic research is commonly appropriate to consider. That the model is log-linear implies no inherent restriction on the form of the occurrence relation – how the rate, or the rate ratio, is a function of age, for example. Insofar as such a model actually is well designed (as to the form of the occurrence relation in its referent domain), including sufficiency of the built-in conditionality of the rate's relation (descriptive) to the risk factor at issue, the modeling provides ready definition of the critically relevant RR^* (addressed above and in sect. 4.3).

Thus far the focus here has been on models in the context of an all-or-none index history. This needs to be supplemented by consideration of the more general case in which

$$X_1 = \text{history score (numerical, ordinal)},$$

so that index histories involve $X_1 > 0$ with $X_2 = 0$ and the reference history is represented by $X_1 = X_2 = 0$. Now the interest is in results specific to non-zero values of X_1, and corresponding to the ith non-zero category the fitted function is evaluated at $X_1 = i$ and $X_2 = 0$ to derive the corresponding $RR_i^* = O_i/\hat{E}_i$ (cf. sect. 4.2).

As we noted at the end of section 4.3 above, modeling of the occurrence relation and study of the relevant parameters imbedded in the model does away with the problems that characterize the needed conditioning when adjusting R_0 to R_0^* in the framework of cross-stratification, especially when the number of strata is quite large. For there is no feasibility problem and not much loss of efficiency in the study of RR^* in consequence of inclusion of added potential confounders into the model. But this adduces a new problem: uncertainty about the adequacy of the model in providing the intended conditioning of the rate's (descriptive) relation to the risk factor at issue. The solution is devoid of the desired 'feel for the data.'

With all this said about the designed object of an etiogenetic epidemiological study, it may be appropriate to recall one of the most important contributions of Immanuel Kant into scientific thought. He taught that it is not a scientist's role to simply read the Book of Nature, by accruing experience in such terms as it happens to present itself. Instead, (s)he is to define, before whatever research experience, the terms in which (s)he needs to 'consult' Nature. In epidemiological research, the *form* of the occurrence relation at issue – defining the object(s) of study – is to be defined before actually having the experience, and the role of the research experience is, merely, to supply empirical *content* of that preset form.

The deployment of modeling is generally necessary in (non-experimental) etiogenetic research but that uncertainty about the model's adequacy in providing for the intended conditionality and that lack of 'feel for the data' can be overcome. See section 5.4.

Chapter 5
Etiologic Studies' Essentials

Abstract Given that a defined *study base* is a sine-qua-non for any admissible type of etiogenetic study, and that each person-moment in it is to represent the domain of the designed model for the cases' rate of occurrence, it generally cannot be operationally formed, nor even directly defined; it must be defined as a segment of the population-time within a defined source population-time, a *source base*. The latter, in turn, is formed by the course of a defined source population over a particular span of time, with this population possibly defined indirectly, as the catchment population (of cases) secondary to the directly-defined manner of case identification.

Cases of the outcome event are identified, comprehensively, in the source-base experience, and a fair sample of the source base (of the infinite number of person-moments constituting it) is drawn. The resulting first-stage case and base series are reduced to instances from the actual study base (as defined), to the actual pair of *study series*.

The model – log-linear – for the cases' rate of occurrence implies its corresponding *logistic* model to be fitted to the data (with $Y = 1$ and $Y = 0$ for the case and base series, respectively), yielding a result for the rate ratio of interest, as a function of the modifiers of this as they are accounted for in the model. This, in turn, provides for calculation of the 'expected' number of index cases in the calculation of the essential result, that for the factor-conditional etiogenetic proportion.

These calculations under the designed model lack the intuitive appeal of those based on cross-stratification of the data according to the confounders being controlled. A solution to this problem is *stratification by a unidimensional confounder score*, provided by the fitted logistic function evaluated at the reference category of the etiogenetic determinant under study. Examination of the data in these strata allows verification of freedom from confounding by the extraneous determinants accounted for, and the calculation of the desired result is intuitive and straightforward.

5.1   Source Base, Study Base

Whereas the designed form of an occurrence relation – for the (rate of) occurrence of the illness at issue in a defined domain – defines the object parameters for an etiologic/etiogenetic study, and whereas an actual study of that occurrence relation (of the object parameters in it) is to document experience of that form, the first-order topic in the design of an actual etiogenetic study is selection of a particular experience for that documentation.

The end result of this selection – the adopted *study base* – usually is an aggregate of *population-time* from the designed occurrence relation's domain, for documentation of *incidence density* (of an event-type outcome), the dependence of this rate on the determinants of it in the form of the predesigned occurrence relation. The person-moments in this study base (infinite in number) represent the designed occurrence relation's defined domain (for the outcome's occurrence), and associated with each of these person-moments is an/the index history or the reference history, or, perhaps, some 'other' history. Besides, the person-moments constituting the study base may have been designed to satisfy various admissibility criteria of a purely practical sort – the person at the time being compos mentis and fluent in a particular language, for example.

A study base of this type is defined in stages. Defined before the study base itself is the *source base*, and the study base proper is then defined by applying the admissibility criteria to the person-moments constituting the source base. The source base also is defined in two stages. The first stage is the selection of – and commitment to – a particular *source population*.

The definition of the source population may be direct – that of the resident population of a particular metropolitan area or the prescribers to a particular health-insurance plan, for example. Alternatively, direct – primary – definition may be given to the scheme of identification of cases of the illness/outcome at issue, which makes the source population to have an indirect definition secondary to this: it gets to be the *catchment population* of this scheme – the entirety of those who, at any given moment, are in the 'were-would' state of: were the outcome event (clinical inception of the illness) now to occur, the case would be 'caught' by that scheme.

With the source population defined, the actual source base for an etiogenetic study of incidence density (in causal relation to histories in respect to the risk factor at issue) needs further definition, in terms of time. For dynamic source populations (being open for exit, and hence having turnover of membership), such as the residents of a particular metropolitan area, the source base is generally defined as the source population's course over an interval in calendar time. The same can be true of a source base formed from a previously formed, multipurpose, cohort-type source population (which is closed for exit, even by death). But if the source population is a cohort formed ad hoc, then the members' contributions to the population-time of the source base are prone to start from their enrollments into the cohort, at different points in calendar time, but end simultaneously in calendar time if not earlier, due to death or loss to follow-up.

Given the source base for an etiogenetic study of the usual type, dealing with incidence density, the actual study base within it indeed is merely defined, not formed by any process of admissions (of person-moments) into it. The study population generally is dynamic even if the source population is a cohort: a person's contribution to the population-time of the study base begins when admissibility to it first gets to be satisfied, and it ends when those criteria no longer are satisfied; the study population thereby has turnover of membership (which here is the meaning of 'dynamic').

Exceptionally, the study base is one for a *proportion-type rate*, and so therefore also is the source base in which this is imbedded. Both of these are constituted by a *series of person-moments*, a finite – 'enumerable' – series, instead of an aggregate of population-time (constituted by an infinite number of person-moments).

5.2 Case Series, Base Series

As the empirical occurrence relation being documented in an etiologic/etiogenetic study addresses the outcome's occurrence in the study base – the rate of this occurrence as a function of its determinants – the study inescapably needs to involve, for one, identification of the cases of the outcome that occur in the study base; it needs to produce the *case series* that supplies the numerator inputs into the empirical rates being documented (sect. 4.2).

Cases of the outcome are first identified in the source base, and this first-stage case series then is to be reduced to what ultimately is needed: the series of cases occurring in the actual study base – their associated person-moments satisfying the criteria of a person-moment's admissibility into the study base (sect. 5.1 above). For reasons of validity assurance the aim generally is to identify all of these cases, even though an assuredly fair – stochastically representative – sample also would be consistent with validity assurance. After all, an etiogenetic study ultimately is about rate ratios, not absolute rates (sects. 4.2, 4.3, 4.4).

It bears emphasis that not only is a series of cases of the outcome at issue a sine-qua-non element in the structure of an etiogenetic study, but the role of this case series is to provide numerator inputs into (the calculation of empirical) *rates* in a defined experience of the outcome's occurrence – in the *study base* (sect. 4.2).

The *'case-control'* study (sect. 6.2), while still commonly deployed (ch. 2), represents a notable failure to appreciate this role of the case series in a rational etiogenetic study. A case series without a defined experience of case occurrence as its referent is not a case series of a rational etiogenetic study, as this case series isn't in the role of providing numerator inputs into rates (empirical; sect. 4.2).

More to this same effect: If one were to specify the single most basic element – the single most fundamental sine-qua-non – in the structure of an etiogenetic study, one would have to assign this status to the expressly defined study base. This point bears emphasis because of the still-common adherence to that 'case-control' study concept (that 'trohoc' fallacy; sect. 6.2).

Given the study base and the case series providing numerator inputs into (quantification of) the outcome's index and reference rates of occurrence in this study base, obviously needed also is a source of the corresponding denominator inputs; that is, needed also is a *base series* to accompany that case series, to provide denominator inputs into (the documentation of) the ratio of the index and reference rates in the study base.

When, as is usual, the study base is an aggregate of population-time (for study of incidence density), the base series necessarily is a *sample* of the study base (as the population-time of it is constituted by an infinite number of person-moments). As a sample – a stochastically representative one – the base series provides numbers (tallies) proportional (stochastically) to the population-time referents of the rates of comparative concern; and proportionality in this sense is all that is needed, as the etiogenetic interest is not in rates per se but only in their ratios (sects. 4.2, 4.3, 4.4).

When the study base is a series (enumerable, finite) of person-moments, census of it for the base series always is an option in principle; but it may not be justifiable on the ground of its inefficiency. Census may be unjustifiable if, in a study of a proportion-type rate, there is a procedural distinction between the acquisition of the case series and that of the base series. But there may be but a single series of the person-moments constituting the study base, with the case series identifiable only as a subset in this base series.

A base series is to represent the study base at large, and not merely of that segment of the base in which a case of the outcome is not associated with the person-moment. When the study base is one of population-time, a sample (finite) of it (of the infinite number of person-moments in it) is not expected to include any instances in which the outcome event is associated with a person-moment in the sample. But in a sample – and especially in a census – of a study base constituted by a series (finite) of person-moments, instances of the outcome can be involved in the base series – and to the extent they are, they belong there.

5.3   Model Fitting, Study Result

The two series from the study base – the case series and the base series – naturally are documented in respect to everything that is involved in the designed occurrence relation. And whatever may be the format of the primary documentation of those data and the codings applied to these, in the end the data are in the form of *realizations of the statistical variates* in the designed occurrence relation. In these terms there is a *data matrix* with columns for Y, X_1, X_2, etc., where $Y = 1$ and $Y = 0$ indicate the presence and the absence, respectively, of a case of the outcome at issue (i.e., membership of the instance – the person-moment – in the case or the base series).

In the usual situation in which the designed model addresses *incidence density*, fitted to the data is the *logistic* counterpart of that model:

$$\log\left[\Pr\left(Y = 1\right) / \Pr\left(Y = 0\right)\right] = B_0 + \sum\nolimits_k B_k X_k.$$

The 'intercept' (B_0) in this reflects, in part, the chosen size of the base series relative to that of the case series; but the rest of the parameters are, quantitatively, the same as in the designed occurrence relation – including, of course, the subset of those parameters constituting the actual objects of the study (sect. 4.4).

More directly relevant for the knowledge-base of etiognosis about the rate of morbidity is a result secondary to this direct one. The study produced an 'observed' number of cases of the outcome in association with the ith index history for the etiogenetic determinant (of the outcome's rate of occurrence). This observed number ($O_i = C_i$) divided by an 'estimate' ($\hat{E}_i$) of the corresponding 'expected' number equals the crude overall index rate (R_i) divided by the overall reference rate adjusted to the structure of R_i:

$$C_i/\hat{E}_i = R_i/R_0^* = \widehat{RR}_i^*$$

(sect. 4.3). This is the empirical counterpart (from the study at issue) of the RR that determines the factor-conditional etiogenetic proportion (among the $O = C_1$ cases): $(RR_i^* - 1)/RR_i^*$ (sect. 4.3).

The *model-fitting counterpart* of this RR* is

$$\widehat{RR}_i^* = C_i/\sum_j (1/RR_{ij}),$$

where the RR_{ij} set corresponds to the C_i set: it is the set of RR values from the study-produced RR function corresponding to (the profiles of) the C_i subset of cases, and the summation is over the members of the C_i set (sects. 4.3, 4.4).

If at issue is a proportion-type rate on the basis of an enumerable (finite) set of person-moments, the designed log-linear model (sect. 4.2) is fitted to the data (possibly a single series) as such; and the results for the RR function, $\widehat{RR}^*$, and the factor-conditional etiogenetic proportion flow from this quite analogously with those having to do with incidence density (above).

With that $\widehat{RR}_i^*$ set ($i = 1, 2, \ldots$) the principal results of the study, their *precisions* need to be quantified (incl. for the purposes of its synthesis with the corresponding results from other studies), perhaps best in terms of their associated 95% 'confidence' intervals. That interval implies its counterpart for the factor-conditional etiogenetic proportion of interest.

A simple way to accomplish this begins with fitting a model involving separate indicators for the index histories with no product terms based on these and noting the fitted value of each of the corresponding parameters ($\hat{B}$) together with its SE ('standard error'). Then, a 95% interval for the logarithm of RR*$_i$ can be derived as

$$\left[\log\left(\widehat{RR}_i^*\right)\right](1 \pm 2.0/w),$$

where w is the realization of the 'Wald statistic' – that 'point estimate' of the 'coefficient,' $\hat{B}$, divided by its SE. This has an obvious counterpart for the overall $\widehat{RR}^*$.

Deriving the $\widehat{RR}^*$ and a measure of precision of this is reasonable to do even when the study is one of *hypothesis testing* about the very existence of the etiogenetic connection, and not yet a study on the magnitude of an established etiogenetic connection. For, the magnitude of the empirical $\widehat{RR}^*$ is informative for this qualitative purpose together with the null P-value (from that Wald statistic, perhaps). For synthesis of the result with those of other studies, relevant is the fitted logistic function together with the SEs of the relevant coefficients in it.

5.4   Demystifying the Modeling

Any serious etiogenetic research is characterized by the resulting rate ratio's – $\widehat{RR}^*$'s – conditionality on a reasonably complete set of extraneous determinants (of the magnitude) of the reference rate. This generally means that the traditional cross-stratification approach to the conditioning – with its propensity to 'break down' in the context of multiple dimensions in the cross-stratification – is now commonly replaced by the modeling approach (sect. 4.4). But the ideal approach arguably is one which captures the virtues of each of those two approaches while avoiding the drawbacks of each of them.

Given a history of the all-or-none type, the notation for the frequencies in the j-th stratum in cross-stratification (by gender, categories of age, etc.) could be taken to be this:

	$D = 1$	$D = 0$	Total
	c_{1j}	c_{0j}	C_j
	b_{1j}	b_{0j}	B_j

where the sizes of the subsets for this stratum of the overall case series (of size C) and base series (of size B) are C_j and B_j, respectively; and of these, the further subsets from the etiogenetic determinant's index category ($D = 1$) and reference category ($D = 0$) are of sizes c_{1j} and c_{0j} from the C_j, and b_{1j} and b_{0j} from the B_j.

The set of J tables like this gives the centrally relevant parameter – the $\widehat{RR}^*$ determining the factor-conditional etiogenetic proportion (sect. 5.3 above) – the empirical value

$$\widehat{RR}^* = C_1/\hat{E}_1 = C_1/\sum_j \hat{E}_{ij}$$

$$= \sum_j c_{1j}/\sum_j \left(c_{1j}/\widehat{RR}_j\right)$$

$$= \sum_j c_{1j}/\sum_j \left\{c_{1j}/\left[(c_{1j}/b_{1j})/(c_{0j}/b_{0j})\right]\right\}$$

$$= \sum_j c_{1j}/\sum_j (b_{1j}c_{0j}/b_{0j}).$$

The inefficiency – and its consequent instability, imprecision – of this measure arises from the susceptibility of those $\hat{E}_j$ values to considerable chance variation, notably when the data from some of the strata are quite sparse. A remedy to this is, in principle, reduction of the number of the strata – by pooling pairs or larger subsets of the strata, so long as this is reasonably consistent with maintaining the intended conditionality on the stratification factors. If such pooling, consistent with retention of the conditionality, leads to quite small a number of strata, then quite good efficiency is achieved, after all.

The necessary condition for the poolability – 'collapsibility' – of two or more strata is (near-)constancy of the theoretical value corresponding to either the c_{0j}/b_{0j} or the b_{1j}/b_{0j} ratio – that is, of the theoretical (quasi-)rate of the outcome's occurrence conditional on the object determinant's reference category *or* of the ratio of the sizes of the index and reference subsegments of the study base across strata at issue.

This leads to consideration of replacement of cross-stratification of the data by *uni-dimensional stratification* for the same purpose – stratification by a *scoring function* such as is involved, for the needed conditioning, in the modeling alternative to the cross-stratification. The modeling ordinarily addresses the outcome's occurrence; but it could address, for the conditioning purpose at issue here, the study determinant's distribution in the study base (the relative sizes of the $D = 1$ and $D = 0$ segments of it).

This hybrid of the traditional cross-stratification approach and its modern model-based alternative retains the merits of both of these – without introducing material problems of its own. It retains the ready intelligibility of the stratification approach – its associated real 'feel for the data' – while it also exploits the efficiency – and hence the feasibility of truly multi-dimensional conditioning – characterizing the modeling approach.

The scoring function, when used for conditioning in the meaning of equalization of the 'background' risks for the contrast at issue, is the fitted regression function evaluated at the focal determinant's reference category (at $D = 0$). With the value of this function calculated for each of the data points (person-moments) in the database and the strata (of risk) formed on this basis, the first concern should generally be to verify – and document for the study report – the expected: that each of the extraneous determinants (of the outcome's rate of occurrence) indeed has, within each of the strata, a suitably balanced distribution between the index ($D = 1$) and reference ($D = 0$) segments of the base series.

Upon these preparatory steps, the production of the actual main result – the value of $(C_1/\hat{E}_1)$ or $\widehat{RR}^*$ – proceeds as outlined above. And the precision of this result can quantified as outlined in section 5.3.

Chapter 6
Etiologic Studies' Typology

Abstract It remains commonplace to think of *design options* for etiogenetic studies in terms of 'cohort' and 'case-control' studies, first and foremost. But it should be understood that the essential features of etiogenetic studies are not optional. These are features logically deduced from correct conception of what etiogenesis, as a genre of causation, actually is (chap. 3 Abstract), and they are: study base representing the designed (sub)domain of the cases' occurrence, case series and a sample from this study base, etc (chaps. 4, 5 Abstracts). And it should be understood that the 'cohort' and 'case-control' studies, for example, do not satisfy the logical requirements for an etiogenetic study.

We think of these purported design options as the *cohort fallacy* and the *trohoc fallacy*, respectively, and we present the necessary corrections of each of them. We also consider two other purported design options for etiogenetic studies, redefining one and correcting the other. From the different points of departure we thus forge unity: *E pluribus unum* (à la seal of the U.S.), namely *the* etiogenetic study.

In the framework of the a-priori, singular nature of the etiogenetic study there remain *true design options* in various aspects of it. The source population can be defined either directly or indirectly (as the cases' catchment population); and if it is defined directly, it may be defined as a cohort or as a dynamic population. The source population/base can be 'monolithic' or fragmented/scattered. The case identification in the source base can be directed to all cases of the illness at issue or, for reasons of validity assurance, to cases that are severe but otherwise typical in their manifestations. The sampling of the source base can be indiscriminate or, for efficiency enhancement, suitably stratified. Etc. In this way, the singular nature of the logically tenable type of etiogenetic study leaves open a multitude of design options: *E unum pluribus*.

6.1 Cohort Study: Its Essence – Corrected

In epidemiological usage, '*cohort*' should be understood to mean a population that is *closed*, specifically closed for *exits*: once a member, always a member. Thus, membership in the cohort deployed for all the studies in the framework of the famous *Framingham Heart Study* – misnomer for cardiovascular disease research program founded on a source cohort recruited from the town of Framingham in Massachusetts – has not undergone any attrition, not even on the basis of the original members' deaths. Even though practically all of this cohort's members already are deceased, they still constitute an undiminished source population for studies – on the basis of the *in vivo* data on them. The collection of all of the data was once prospective ($T > T_0$) in cohort time but it always was, and still is, retrospective ($T < T_0$) in any study time of exploiting the data.

The nature of the resident population of the town of Framingham, from which the cohort was recruited, is different. This population is *open* for exits, for terminations of membership – by death, for example. As a consequence of the exits in conjunction with new entries, this population has turnover of membership; it is a *dynamic* population in this sense. The FHS could have been constructed in the framework of this resident population of the town, as such, as its source population. Like the cohort recruited from it, this dynamic population could have been subjected to biennial surveys for routine data collection. The actual FHS cohort, as it got to be documented, would now be identifiable from the database that could have been produced from this dynamic source population.

What in etiologic/etiogenetic research is now routinely termed *cohort study* used to be known as *prospective* study (and also as *follow-up* study), distinguishing it from what was termed retrospective study (and alternatively case history study); but the 'prospective-study' precursor of the 'cohort-study' term was discarded on the ground that its antonym got to be viewed as unduly denigrating of the perceived alternative to it, now known by the higher-sounding name case-control study.

In a cohort study (so-called, in etiogenetic research), a cohort-type study population is recruited from the chosen source population (cohort-type or dynamic). As of the time of the enrollments (at $T = 0$ on the scale of cohort time) the members of this cohort are documented in relevant respects, most notably as to their histories in respect to the etiogenetic determinant at issue. The members are then followed (into prospective cohort time) to document the occurrence/non-occurrence of the illness whose etiogenesis is being studied. And the thus-accrued data are 'analysed' (meaning synthesized) to express how the outcome's occurrence was related to the divergence in the causal determinant (with certain conditionings in this; cf. sect. 4.4) – the outcome prospective and the determinant retrospective on the scale of cohort time.

The idea in the genesis of the 'cohort' study (on etiogenesis) was to emulate the intervention-prognostic experiment, the *intervention trial* (clinical); but in such a trial the outcome's prospective occurrence is related to prospective (*sic*) divergence in the causal determinant (the interventions), both of these in cohort time. On this basis already, *this paradigm was ill-chosen* – without appreciation of the profound difference between etiogenetic and interventive causations, at issue in etiognosis and intervention-prognosis, respectively (sect. 3.1).

The genuine essentials of an etiogenetic study flow directly from the nature of this genre of causation (sects. 3.1, 4.2; ch. 5), with no paradigmatic role for the intervention trial in this. And as for etiogenetic causation, critically important to appreciate is its retrospective nature, from the vantage of time of the outcome's occurrence/non-occurrence (at – in association with – a particular person-moment; sect. 5.1). For this reason and in this sense, *any etiogenetic study is to be thought of as inherently being a retrospective study* (while any intervention-prognostic study inherently is a prospective study; ch. 9).

Given that in a 'cohort' study (on etiogenesis) the causal histories are documented as of the enrollments into the study cohort – so that the T_0 of etiogenetic time is made to coincide with the T_0 of cohort time – the outcome theoretically ought to be ascertained at this same point in time; but this *theoretically correct 'cohort' study is impracticable*, as an infinite number of these person-moments would be required (as the requisite size of the cohort $\rightarrow \infty$ as duration of follow-up $\rightarrow 0$).

Insofar as a cohort's follow-up – inherently prospective in cohort time – indeed is to be taken as definitional to 'cohort' studies (on etiogenesis), important *corrections* in the rest of the concept – the 'cohort fallacy' – need to be made. The cohort must be seen to be (not the study cohort but) only the source cohort; and its follow-up must be seen to be (not merely the means to identify the outcome events but) the formation of the source base, from which to identify the first-stage case series and to draw a suitable first-stage base series, etc. – as outlined in chapter 5 above.

Upon these corrections, the concept of 'cohort' study is none other than that of a first-principles etiogenetic study in the framework of a cohort-type source population. This cohort feature of the study, in itself, is of no quality consequence to the study, which actually involves a dynamic study population forming the study base (sect. 5.1). It is consequential only if the cohort's follow-up was/is used to document the etiogenetic histories before the person-moments in the case and base series, and if this is materially relevant to the validity of these histories.

6.2 Case-control Study: Its Essence – Corrected

A 'cohort' study, as it has been construed, is prone to be quite onerous to carry out. In order that the cohort's follow-up yield a reasonably large number of the outcome events, needed generally is the enrollment – and at-enrollment documentation – of quite a large cohort and its follow-up for quite a long time. "The main feature of a cohort study," says the I.E.A. Dictionary of Epidemiology (specified in sect. 3.2), "is observation of large numbers over a long period (commonly years) ..."

Much more practical is a study that, instead of the enrollment and follow-up of a cohort, begins with a case series; and especially, if it ends with that series. "Fritz Lickint in 1929 was the first to publish statistical evidence joining lung cancer and cigarettes [ref.]. ... His evidence was fairly simple, constituting what epidemiologists today call a *'case series'* showing that lung cancer patients were particularly likely to be smokers. ... Franz H. Müller [in his] 1939 medical dissertation [ref.] presents the world's first controlled epidemiological study of the tobacco-lung cancer relationship, ... His analysis was what we today would call a ... *case-control study*, meaning that he compared ... the smoking behavior of lung cancer patients with that of a healthy 'control group' of comparable age" (ref. below; italics ours). Müller did not have to enroll and document a large cohort, and then to follow it for years, to get his documented 86 'cases' and 86 'controls.'

Reference: Proctor RN. *The Nazi War on Cancer*. Princeton: Princeton University Press, 1999; pp. 183, 194-96.

Relative to the 'cohort' study (in its uncorrected form), the 'case-control' study (also in its uncorrected form; above) has, apart from its practicality, the theoretical virtue that the causal histories are specified on a scale of (retrospective) time whose T_0 is the time of outcome – on the scale of the relevant, etiogenetic time.

On the other hand, though, while the 'cohort' study has a study base of sorts (the series of person-moments of enrollment into the cohort), *the 'case-control' study is devoid of any inherent referent for its result in the form of study base.* The result's referent is a 'case group' together with its 'control group' (cf. above). There thus is no inherent specification of a population-time, or of a series (finite, enumerable) of person-moments, for which rates – or rate ratios – are documented. And as there is no inherent conception of study base as the referent of the study result, there is *no base series* to supplement the case series, to provide information about the denominator inputs into the compared rates. The 'case-control' study is, thus, grossly at variance with the essentials of etiogenetic studies set forth in sections 5.1 and 5.2. Seen to represent the reverse of the 'cohort' study, it has been alternatively termed the 'trohoc' study ('trohoc' being the heteropalindrome of 'cohort'); and the profound fallacy in it may thus be termed the 'trohoc fallacy.'

As the comparison of the index and reference rates of the outcome's occurrence in a defined study base is replaced by comparison of 'cases' with 'controls,' which comparison does not correspond to the causal contrast (cause present vs. its defined alternative present, in the study base), strange things happen – things that should have been interpreted as indicating that the comparison is anomalous. One of these is the phenomenon of '*overmatching*,' which is prone to occur in 'case-control' studies but not in 'cohort' studies. Had Müller in his 'case-control' study (above) matched his 'controls' to his 'cases' according to some close correlate of smoking (such as habitual match-carrying), the distribution of his 'controls' by smoking history would have been very similar to that of his 'cases,' while no matching of non-smokers to smokers, by whatever correlate of smoking, in a 'cohort' study would have the corresponding consequence in respect to their relative rates of subsequent occurrence of lung cancer.

Closely related to this anomalous consequence of matching in 'case-control' studies is another one. Matching of the 'controls' to the 'cases' in these studies has commonly been thought of as being a means to prevent confounding. But prevention of confounding (distinct from control of it) can only be a matter of seeing to it that the index and reference segments of the study base have suitably balanced – similar – distributions according to the potential confounder – an extraneous determinant of the outcome's rate of occurrence in the reference segment of the study base (sect. 4.3). And given the absence of study base in the concept, a 'case-control' study *does not provide for detection of actual confounding nor even for meaningful thinking about it* (about this feature of the study base).

The 'case-control' study thus requires a fundamental *correction* in terms of introduction of the ever-necessary concept of study base (sect. 5.2). And secondary to this, it requires the understanding that 'cases' are not a group of people but a series of person-moments with this study base as its referent – by representing the entirety of the cases occurring in it – and that for the 'controls' for it to be meaningful at all, they actually need to constitute a fair sample of this study base, to form a base series in this meaning (cf. sect. 5.2).

The way the cases of the outcome (illness) are identified in a 'case-control' study implies its corresponding *catchment population* as the study's *source population*. This is the population (dynamic) whose membership is defined by the 'were-would' state of: were the outcome event now to occur, it would be 'caught' by the study's case ascertainment scheme (cf. sect. 5.1). This can be the way – indirect – of defining the source population for the etiogenetic study that comes about as a result of the necessary corrections' introduction into the 'case-control' study. For the source base defined by the case ascertainment over a span of time the case ascertainment is complete by definition, and the challenge is fair sampling of that source base for the first-stage base series.

Alternatively, upon the correction, the source population is defined directly (as the adult resident population of a particular metropolitan area, say; sect. 5.1), and complete case ascertainment for the source base is now the challenging part (while fair sampling of it is not).

6.3   Cross-sectional Study: Its Essence – Redefined

Under 'Cross-sectional study,' the I.E.A. dictionary (specified in sect. 3.2) gives this:

> A study that examines the relation between diseases (or other health-related characteristics) and other variables of interest as they exist in a defined population at one particular time. The presence or absence of disease and the presence or absence of the other variables (or, if they are quantitative, their level) are documented in each member of the study population or in a representative sample at one particular time. The relationship between a variable and the disease can be examined (1) in terms of the prevalence of disease in different population subgroups defined according to the presence or absence (or level) of the variables and (2) in terms of the presence or absence (or level) of the variables in the diseases versus the nondiseased. Note that disease prevalence rather than incidence is normally recorded in a cross-sectional study [ref.]. The temporal sequence of cause and effect cannot necessarily be determined in a cross-sectional study.

We suggest that, actually, the essence of the 'cross-sectional' etiogenetic study is, simply, this: The study base is formed as a *single series* of person-moments, as in a 'cohort' study, but outcomes associated with these person-moments are ascertained with *no follow-up* – the outcome being presence/absence of *prevalent case* of the illness at those person-moments.

'Cross-sectional' study is rather commonly presented as one element in the triad in which the other elements are 'cohort' study and 'case-control' study, but as the least eminent element in this triad. As we define it (above), it is distinguished from 'cohort' study by the absence of follow-up (for outcome determinations); and the absence of (distinctly) separate formations of the 'case group' and the 'control group' distinguishes it from 'case-control' study.

Absence of follow-up means that 'cross-sectional' study is *not 'longitudinal'* in time (diachronic) in the meaning that 'cohort' study inherently is (by the follow-up in it); but it is just as amenable to consideration of longitudinal histories as 'cohort' study (and 'case-control' study also) is. Thus the meaning of 'cross-sectional' here is not that the outcome-determinant relation is non-longitudinal (synchronic) by definition, nor do the person-moments constituting the study base inherently represent a cross-section of the source population at a particular point in calendar time or on any other scale of time. In this meaning (cf. quote above), the term is a plain *misnomer*.

Because of the absence of follow-up, the person-moments constituting the study base are classified as of those very moments as for the occurrence – then presence/absence – of the outcome at issue; and at issue thus inherently is, as we put forward in the definition above, an outcome state (rather than event). Its occurrence therefore is documented in terms of its rate of prevalence – this, naturally again, in relation to the etiogenetic factor, conditionally on extraneous determinants of the outcome's prevalence (in the defined domain of study, represented by each of the person-moments constituting the study base).

When the designed occurrence relation (incorporating the object parameter[s] for the study) addresses prevalence (of a state-type outcome), a single series of person-moments obviously is an admissible option for the *study base*. And in the framework of this option, a subset of this series constitutes the *case series* for the study, while the series in its totality can serve as the *base series* – with sampling of that study base an available option for the latter (sect. 5.2).

With this conception of the essence of the 'cross-sectional' etiogenetic study and this understanding of the implications of this essence, this least eminent member of the purported triad of fundamental types of etiogenetic study is one of major distinction: Different from the 'cohort' study and the 'case-control' study, the definitional essence of the 'cross-sectional' study embodies *no need for corrections* – upon the necessary correction of the definition of its essence.

6.4   Semi-cohort Study: Its Essence – Corrected

As we noted in section 1.1, epidemiological practice has been particularly eminent in *occupational* medicine, and so consequently also has been epidemiological research for this discipline of medicine. The generic aim of this research has been the identification of health hazards relatively common in, if not specific to, work environments (as the basis for illness-preventive actions in occupational settings).

A common type of etiologic/etiogenetic study on incidence in this framework has been one that is neither 'cohort' nor 'case-control' study but something that might be termed *semi-cohort study*, as it involves an index cohort but no reference cohort: A cohort of workers representing, at its enrollment, the index category of the hypothesized etiogenetic determinant for a particular illness – typical has been exposure to a potentially carcinogenetic airborne substance in the etiogenesis of lung cancer – is recruited and suitably documented at enrollment. It is followed to identify and document occurrences of the outcome – say deaths from lung cancer as proxies for clinical inceptions of the disease. A given number of these events is 'observed' in the course of the cohort's follow-up, and the corresponding 'expected' number in derived by applying the local or national 'general population' rates of the event's occurrence, specific for gender and age, to the various gender-age strata of the cohort's follow-up time. The thus-derived $O/\hat{E}$ ratio is the 'standardized mortality (or morbidity) ratio,' SMR, result of the study (cf. sect. 4.3).

For this quite primitive study – well recognized to be marred by the 'healthy worker effect' – an *improved* counterpart – free of that anomalous 'effect' – would have as its source population the union of two cohorts: such an 'index' cohort together with a 'reference' cohort of workers who at cohort T_0 represent not only the determinant's reference category but also similar occupational exposure, pre- and post-T_0, to extraneous causes of the outcome and, just as importantly, similar distributions by other unquantifiable extraneous determinants of the outcome's rate of occurrence (e.g., socio-economic status, if relevant). With the source base thus formed – as the union of the two cohorts' population-time of follow-up – the rest of the elements of a *first-principles etiogenetic study* flow from it: the source base; the first-stage case and base series; the reduced, second-stage counterparts of these; etc. (ch. 5). The etiogenetic histories in this corrected counterpart of the semi-cohort study are not defined as of cohort T_0 – any more than in the corrected counterpart of the 'cohort' – 'full-cohort' – study.

6.5 *E Pluribus Unum*

As it is at present, design of an etiologic/etiogenetic study is thought fundamentally to involve the choice among 'cohort' study, 'case-control' study, and 'cross-sectional' study in the main, with the understanding that there also are some other fundamental options to consider (such as the 'semi-cohort' study; sect. 6.4 above).

But implicit in the foregoing in this chapter is the idea that the principal ones among these purported fundamental options – the 'cohort' study and the 'case-control' study – are logically inadmissible (sects. 6.1, 6.2) and that the 'cross-sectional' study, while logically admissible, has a raison d'être only when the outcome phenomenon is a state (sect. 6.3), while it ordinarily is an event (sects. 6.1, 6.2, 6.3).

In the spirit of the Latin words in seal of the U.S., implicit in the foregoing is the idea that a wholesome *unum*/unity can be forged from the now-perceived *pluribus*/variety of principal types of etiogenetic study; that a certain fundamental unity is inherent in the logically admissible types of population-level non-experimental study on the etiogenesis of an illness; that this unity is to be understood to be in the nature of those studies a priori and not as a consequence of judgements and their consequent decisions in the designs of the studies; that one is to know what features an etiogenetic study inherently has, before setting out to design its particulars in this a-priori framework of inescapable essentials of it.

And to say it again, *a first-principles non-experimental etiogenetic study inherently has these core features:*

1. There is an expressly defined *study base*, each of the person-moments in it representing the designed occurrence relation's domain (abstract) and also consistency with whatever pragmatic admissibility criteria besides.
2. There is a case series identified from the study base, intended to be representative of all of the cases of the outcome phenomenon occurring in the study base; that is, having the study base as its referent in this meaning.
3. There is a base series as a fair sample of the study base; that is, a series having, in this sense, the study base as its referent (the study base being, a priori, the referent of the study result).
4. The elements (person-moments) in the case series and base series are documented in all relevant respects, that is, not only as to the series identification (case series vs. base series) but also as to histories in respect to the determinant at issue (generally on a scale with T_0 the time of the person-moment in the series), the confounders in the designed occurrence relation, and such modifiers of the rate ratio as were designed into the occurrence relation defining the objects of the study.
5. From these data is deduced (synthesized) the empirical rate-ratio for the outcome's occurrence (in the study base), index category versus reference category, conditional on the potential confounders, specifically the confounder-conditional rate ratio in the meaning of the 'observed-to-expected' ratio that determines the empirical value for the factor-conditional etiogenetic proportion.

6.6 *E Unum Pluribus*

Even though the essence of etiologic/etiogenetic type of causation (sect. 3.1) logically implies a fundamental unitarity/singularity in the nature of all first-principles etiogenetic studies (sect. 6.5 above) – a set of features that an etiogenetic study should be understood to have a priori and not as results of ad-hoc decisions in study design – there nevertheless remains a multitude of genuine *design options* in this a-priori framework of unitarity.

These options do not imply a typology of the studies as studies per se (à la 'cohort' study, etc.) but options in the design in respect to only *particular aspects* of the fundamentally singular type of etiogenetic study. And the genuine options

in any given aspect of an etiogenetic represent *logical alternatives* to each other –
as would be cohort study versus dynamic-population study, cross-sectional study
versus longitudinal study, and case-control study vs. cases-alone study, were one
to continue classification of studies themselves according to select aspects of them,
considered in isolation. (A car with automatic transmission is not classified as – and
said to be – an automatic car; and a car with four-wheel drive is not seen to be an
alternative to it. Its logical alternative is understood to be a car with a non-automatic
transmission; but even more is understood, namely that at issue really is not types
of car but of transmission in cars.)

Examples of the design options in etiogenetic studies follow, some of them
harkening back to the study's objects design, others pertaining to its methods
design:

- Outcome: event versus state (e.g., clinical inception vs. subclinical presence)
- Outcome: any case versus select subtype of case
- Source population: cohort-type versus dynamic
- Source population: direct definition versus indirect definition (as catchment
  population)
- Source base: prospective versus retrospective in study time (in which T_0 is the
  time of the study's inception)
- Base sampling: statistical (using sampling frame) versus using extraneous out-
  comes
- Base sampling: indiscriminate ('unmatched') versus discriminate (matched or
  otherwise stratified)
- Etiogenetic histories: recorded before outcome versus ascertained after outcome
  (in case and base series)
- Confounding: prevention versus control (upon documentation)
- Control of confounding: standardization versus modeling versus hybrid of these
  (sect. 5.4)

Several of those items are, implicitly, specific to etiogenetic studies of the usual,
non-experimental type. As for experimental etiogenetic studies, which are of the
form of intervention studies, suffice it to note here that they inherently involve a
cohort-type study population, study base that is prospective in cohort and study
time, and prevention of confounding at cohort T_0 at least; and that they obviously
lend themselves to identification of the case series directly from the study base and
to statistical sampling of this base for the base series – as well as to pre-outcome
documentation of these two series in respect to the contrasted etiogenetic histories,
inter alia. See section 9.3.

Chapter 7
Etiologic Studies' Objects Design

Abstract One of Immanuel Kant's most seminal teachings was the idea that a scientist does not learn by simply observing, 'reading' Nature; that (s)he learns by *reading into Nature the terms in which (s)he thinks about Nature*. It is in these terms that (s)he, in a study, 'interrogates' Nature – seeks tentative answers to questions (s)he poses.

In respect to population-level etiogenetic research this means that, preparatory to a study, the researchers think, deeply, about the rate of occurrence of a health phenomenon – the event of a cancer becoming clinically manifest, say – in a particular domain – initially defined by a range of age alone, perhaps. And they think about the phenomenon's rate of occurrence in causal relation to something in the people's past – their diets' antioxidant content, perhaps.

With such a sketchy point of departure, the investigators need to proceed to refine their idea, in that example the particular meanings they elect to associate with the generic terms in: the (rate of) occurrence of 'cancer' in causal relation to 'histories' in respect to their diets' 'antioxidant' content, this in a particular 'domain' of the occurrence. They need to decide whether their thinking in this is specific to a particular type of cancer and a particular type of antioxidant, or whether it is generic in one or both of these respects. They need to specify their thinking in respect to the range of time for the etiogenetic role of dietary antioxidants, retrospectively as of the outcome event (its occurrence/non-occurrence). And they need to decide whether the domain of the study is to be age-restricted and one of no previous clinically manifest cancer, for example.

Upon decisions like these, the investigators go on to design a *statistical model* (log-linear) for the outcome's occurrence in the defined domain, with determinants in the form of statistical variates (Xs). The parameters of Nature constituting the *objects of study* are imbedded in this model, the design of this model amounting to the study's *objects design*.

A future with examples like this is envisioned in this chapter. As of now, a study's objects design is not even in the common vocabulary of epidemiological research.

O.S. Miettinen and I. Karp, *Epidemiological Research: An Introduction*,   73
DOI 10.1007/978-94-007-4537-7_7, © Springer Science+Business Media Dordrecht 2012

7.1 Some Considerations in the Design

In epidemiology in the meaning of a discipline of research (sect. 1.3), and in the thinking of epidemiological researchers likewise, there naturally is much concern for the methodology of the studies, of etiologic/etiogenetic studies in particular – for the theory of *methods design* of these studies.

By contrast, and very unjustifiably, *objects design* has not yet become a topic, even, in the theory of etiogenetic research, much less one perceived to also require a theoretical framework. In line with this, while editors of epidemiological journals, like those of other medical journals, expect any study report to include a section on Methods, they generally expect there to be only an Introduction – rather than a section on Objects – immediately in front of this.

As it thus is, the objects of any published etiogenetic study need to be inferred from the *form of the result* (distinct from the empirical content of that form in the result). For to the extent that the design of an etiogenetic study actually does involve – or is preceded by – design of the objects of study, this determines, to the corresponding extent, the form of the result of the study.

Akin to the a-priori singularity in the methodology of etiogenetic studies (sect. 6.5), the object of an etiogenetic study also has a set of generic elements as an *a-priori given*. At issue inherently is the occurrence of a defined phenomenon of health in a defined domain (human), that phenomenon's/outcome's rate of occurrence (momentary, generally incidence density) in that domain in relation to a particular determinant (retrospective) of that rate, its index category or categories relative to its reference category, this relation in terms of rate ratio(s), conditionally on certain extraneous determinants of the outcome's (rate of) occurrence – for causal interpretability of it.

So, the first component topic in an etiogenetic study's objects design naturally is design of the actual *outcome phenomenon* per se, conceptually, usually in the context of its conceptual approximation specified a priori. For example, if the prompting for the study is that evidence from previous research has pointed to the possibility that diets relatively poor in a given antioxidant are etiologic/etiogenetic to a particular type of cancer, while perhaps not to other types of cancer, the first-order object-design question is, whether the outcome phenomenon should be taken to be that cancer, specifically, or whether it should be cancer unspecified (cf. sect. 2.2).

Analogously for the (potentially) *etiogenetic factor*. So if previous research suggests that paucity of a particular antioxidant in the diet is oncogenetic, while some others appear not to be, the corresponding object-design question is, whether the etiogenetic histories should be specific to this particular antioxidant or whether they should, instead, address a suitable overall measure of the diet's antioxidant content (incl. that from dietary supplements; cf. sect. 2.2).

With the outcome and etiogenetic factor designed, the occurrence relation's *domain* – that of the outcome's occurrence, as it will be addressed in the study – becomes a topic in the study's object design. So if the study is about diet deficient in a particular antioxidant, or antioxidants overall, in the etiogenesis of a particular cancer, or cancers overall, the domain design involves consideration of whether childhood should be involved in the domain; and if not, whether the domain should involve restrictions in the adult range of age and in some other respects, such as freedom from any previous overt case of the cancer, or from any cancer, or, even, from other extraneous but potentially oxidation-caused illnesses (notably atheromatotic ones).

With not only the outcome and (potentially) etiogenetic factor but also the study objects' domain specified, the *temporal aspect* of the occurrence relation becomes the topic in the study's object design. The question is, where in time – retrospective from the time of the outcome, the occurrence/non-occurrence of the phenomenon – is the pathogenetic process whose etiogenesis is at issue in the study. Does it take place in, and are the etiogenetically relevant histories correspondingly about, diets prevailing in, say, the last 5 years before the outcome? or are they to be about, say, the first three or four decades of life (with the study domain perhaps about the sixth or seventh decade of life)?

The generally most challenging question remains: what are *all the extraneous determinants* of the outcome's (rate of) occurrence, the distributions of which could confound the study base and, in this case, would call for focus on the occurrence relation conditional on these?

Decisions concerning the study objects' design in the particular example of studying dietary antioxidants in the etiogenesis of cancer obviously have great bearing on the study's methods design and, ultimately, on the meaning of the study's result, the conceptual form of which will be that of the designed object of study (cf. above).

7.2 Some Principles of the Design

The designed form of the object of an etiologic/etiogenetic study represents *particulars* in the framework of the generic form that it, and hence the study result, is to have a priori (sect. 7.1 above). The result of the study will be about the outcome phenomenon's rate of occurrence in the study base, its index segment(s) versus its reference segment, each person-moment in the study base satisfying the criteria for the designed domain of the objects of the study (parameters in the designed occurrence relation) and the empirical rate-ratio being conditional on all of the designed potential confounders.

The result will inherently be *quantitative* – and the magnitude of the empirical rate-ratio matters even when the study is one of hypothesis-testing rather than quantification. And the result will be, inherently, *descriptive* of the particularistic counterpart, in the study base, of the occurrence relation that is designed for its abstract domain.

The intent in the study objects' design – most notably in the way the outcome-antecedent relation is made conditional on extraneous determinants of the outcome's (rate of) occurrence – is that the study result – the empirical occurrence relation – will be informative about the *causal* connection at issue. In reality, however, faulty objects design (just as faulty methods design) can make the study result *misinformative* about the causal connection, about its 'strength' in meaningful terms in a given direction, even apart from the potential incompleteness of its conditionality on all of the potential confounders.

In what follows, we address the principles of an etiogenetic study's objects design in the contexts of two generic examples, very different in kind.

The first example here is about something that we already touched upon in section 2.4 explicitly and in section 7.1 implicitly, namely the etiogenesis of *prostate cancer*. In section 2.4 we quoted from a review of studies – there had been several 'cohort' and 'case-control' studies but no experimental ones – on *dietary fat* in the etiogenesis of this cancer, and here we consider one of each of these two purportedly principal types of etiogenetic study (ch. 6). To these we add a subsequent experimental study on the same factor but in relation to a different cancer. Besides, as for diet deficient in the antioxidant *selenium* in the etiogenesis of prostate cancer, we examine another 'case-control' study and also the experimental study for which it was a partial prompting (there having been no other 'case-control' studies nor any 'cohort' studies before the trial). These five studies are:

1. Shuurman AG et alii. Association of energy and fat intake with prostate carcinoma risk. Results from the Netherlands cohort study. *Cancer* 1999; 86: 1019-27.
2. Hayes RB et alii. Dietary factors and risks for prostate cancer among blacks and whites in the United States. *Cancer Epidemiology, Biomarkers & Prevention* 1999; 8: 25-34.
3. Beresford SAA et alii. Low-fat dietary pattern and risk of colorectal cancer. The Women's Health Initiative Dietary Modification Trial. *JAMA* 2006; 295: 643-54.
4. Yoshizawa K et alii. Study of prediagnostic selenium level in toenails and the risk of advanced prostate cancer. *Journal of the National Cancer Institute* 1998; 90: 1219-24.
5. Lippman SM et alii. Effects of selenium and vitamin E on risk of prostate cancer and other cancers. The Selenium and Vitamin E Cancer Prevention Trial (SELECT). *JAMA* 2009; 301: 39-51.

For broadest orientation here, it needs to be appreciated that, in practically relevant terms, prostate cancer (or any cancer, for that matter) begins with the *inception of sickness* from it (once the cancer becomes overt – clinical – in its progression), and only this event is subject to the formation of the case series in an etiogenetic study. Any study of the etiogenesis of 'prostate cancer' thus must be understood to actually be about the etiogenesis of (the event of) the onset of symptoms and/or signs of it. All five of those studies addressed cancer in the meaning of the event of its clinical inception.

Related to this, and of equally fundamental relevance to the objects design of a study on the etiogenesis of 'cancer' is a duality of phases in the development of symptomatic cancer: the first, *pathogenetic* phase of this (of pathologic changes culminating in the inception of the cancer) is to be distinguished from the second, *progression* phase of it (during the cancer's latent presence). An etiogenetic influence on the pathogenetic phase is termed *initiation* of the cancer, its counterpart in the progression phase being termed *promotion* of the cancer – of its progression. A designed occurrence relation addressing one of these does not thereby also address the other; that is, evidence about one of these (from a given study) is not evidence for or against the other when studying fat-rich or antioxidant-poor diet in the etiogenesis of clinically manifest prostate (or any other) cancer.

The objects design thus needs to be directed, expressly, to the study of initiation or promotion or both, notably because the healthcare implications are very different according to which one of the two phases of the overt cancer's etiogenesis is at issue. Initiation occurs, and initiators thus are to be avoided, in the earliest decades (three or four, say) of life already, while promotion occurs and promoters are to be avoided in middle age and later (as of the fifth decade, say).

This means the need to design the study objects' *domain*, and also the outcome-determinant *temporal relation* in the object, in accordance with whether at issue is initiation or promotion or both in the etiogenesis of the overt form of the cancer (cf. sect. 7.1 above).

All five of those example studies were ones of etiogenetic *hypothesis-testing*, as is quite characteristic of epidemiological research in general (as the research tends to be slow to produce even qualitative knowledge on what it addresses; ch. 2). So, of most fundamental significance to their objects designs was the broadest nature of the hypothesis. Three questions about the hypothesis concerning the etiogenesis of overt cancer are of particular relevance: Is it, as discussed above, about initiation or about promotion of the development of the cancers, or both? Is it, as discussed in section 7.1 above, specific to a particular type of cancer or about cancers quite generally? and, Is it, as also discussed in section 7.1, specific to a particular factor in a given class of them (and its defined alternative) or about a whole class of agents without distinctions among them?

Even though all five of those studies were, as noted above, about the etiogenesis of the inception of the symptomatic stage in the progression of the cancer at issue, none of them was specific, in the study report, on whether the study was about initiation or about promotion of the malignant process, or about both of these, per the nature of the hypothesis.

The determinant histories in those studies, as of the time of outcome, were only about the last few years (rather than decades), as though tested was a hypothesis specifically about *promotion* of the cancer. Yet, the antioxidant hypothesis at least is expressly about the *initiation* of cancer (about diet deficient in antioxidants allowing unopposed accumulation of the oxidative damage to the genome that leads to the development of activated oncogene together with inactivated suppressor gene and, thereby, to initiation of the cancer).

Etiogenetic studies that are insufficiently 'longitudinal' in (the retrospective depth of) their objects are, of course, relatively practicable to carry out; but this flaw in their objects design can be serious to the point of making the study result *misleading*. This problem presumably attends the statement in the PDQ Cancer

Prevention Overview web page of the U.S. National Cancer Institute, that "The results of the [SELECT; ref. 5 above] indicated that taking daily selenium or vitamin E or both did not reduce the incidence of prostate cancer compared with placebo [ref.]." For recruited into that trial were men in their 50s of age or older (rather than young children) and their "median follow-up was 5.46 years" (rather than decades). Thus, by its nature that trial actually was solely about the cancer's promotion, while the hypothesis presumably was about its initiation.

The *principle* that thus was violated in all five of those example studies is this: A meaningfully designed object for an etiogenetic hypothesis-testing study may be infeasible to study (validly); and when it is, it should not be studied through ersatz objects that actually are meaningless in respect to the biological essence of hypothesis. The problem is much worse than futility: it is risking misunderstanding of the study result, not understanding that it is meaningless in respect to the actual hypothesis. It should be understood that some objects of desirable and meaningful epidemiological knowledge are not subject to practicable population-level study; that in respect to them it is necessary to settle for such insights and population-level surmises as can be derived from more 'basic' epidemiological research (cf. sect. 1.2).

Apart from their temporal aspects, the causal contrasts in those five studies, from # 1 to # 5 respectively, were these: a given level of fat intake (kcal/day) vs. another, also conditionally on total energy intake; a given level of foods high in animal fat (grams/day) vs. another, and the same in terms of such foods as a proportion of total energy intake; reductions in fat together with increase in vegetables, fruits, and grains vs. continuation of usual diet; a given level of toenail selenium content vs. another, also conditionally on calcium intake and lycopene intake; and a given level of supplementary antioxidant intake vs. placebo intake.

As in studies # 1 and # 2, meaningful quantification of fat intake indeed is conditional on total energy intake, perhaps expressed as the proportion of the latter. But such quantification remains meaningless except when at issue actually is conditionality on or proportion of total energy intake from fats and, isocalorically, specified alternative nutrients (carbohydrates, most notably), with total energy intake a possible added element in the designed occurrence relation. The contrast in # 3 is a bit of an approximation to what thus is needed, while that in # 4 is sensible, though only isocalorically. Concerning diet supplementation with antioxidants, # 5 is impeccable as for the meaning of the factor contrast (when not considering its temporal aspects).

The *principle* that in this aspect of those example studies' object designs was incompletely heeded is this: While the causal (index) histories in an etiogenetic study are to be explicitly defined and meaningful as such, meaningful explicit definitions also are to be given to the alternative(s) to these. The proper concept of the alternative antecedent – the reference history – in an etiogenetic contrast is not simply absence of the index history at issue.

Concerning the determinant contrast, the example studies considered here raise this question: Insofar as it is reasonable and indeed preferable to study the effect (etiogenetic) of *total fat* content of diet, without distinctions between, say, fats from meats and dairy products as components of this, is it not better, by analogy, to study *total antioxidant* content of diet instead of studying particular components of this? (Cf. sects. 2.2, 7.1.)

And in the same vein, as the fat and antioxidant contents of diet are hypothesized to be etiogenetic to various types of cancer, the question that arises is: Shouldn't the object of study focus on the *cancers unspecified* instead of focusing on a given one of them in any given study? (Cf. sects. 2.2, 7.1.)

The *principle* bearing on answering these two questions is this: Uncalled-for distinction-making among potentially etiogenetic factors and among health outcomes conduces to uncalled-for complexity and its consequent confusion and retardation of progress, and it is, therefore, to be avoided. In those five example studies there generally wasn't even a practical, study-efficiency reason to focus on particular antioxidants or particular cancers instead of composites of these. And, by the way, in studies of smoking in the etiology of cancer, progress would have been even slower than it actually was (sect. 2.7) had distinctions been made among particular brands of cigarette, while the initial focus on cancers of the airways was obviously well-justified (while concern for any cancer, without distinctions, would have further retarded the progress).

A technical problem that attends the focus on a component in a family of conceptually related factors of etiogenetic potential is the need to control all of the others as potential confounders in any non-experimental study on the singled-out component. In the 'case-control' study on selenium level (as measured from toenails) in the etiology of prostate cancer (# 4 above), "lycopene intake" but intake of no other antioxidant was controlled, and the operational meaning of this one type of extraneous antioxidant intake (and "calcium intake" too) was left unspecified.

The *principle* that thus comes to focus is this: In non-experimental testing of an etiogenetic hypothesis, histories of potential confounders need to be conceptualized in truly meaningful terms and accurately documented in these terms (for full control of them). When this is not possible, the object of study needs to be modified to eliminate such a problem – or, the project is to be abandoned altogether. Study of the aggregate intake of antioxidants, without focus on any given one of the components in this, is free of confounding by intakes of extraneous antioxidants. (Different from potential confounders, etiogenetic hypothesis-testing does allow some fuzziness in the histories involved in the causal contrast[s].)

While an etiogenetic study is about the rate of the outcome's occurrence in causal relation to the etiogenetic determinant of this, ultimately in terms of the rate *ratio* for the index category versus reference category contrast(s), those five example studies were quite variable in what their respective results were said to be about. Reported from the 'cohort' study (# 1) was "rate ratio." From the two 'case-control' studies (# 2 and # 4) the results were said to be "odds ratios," and from the two experimental studies (# 3 and # 5) reported were "hazard ratios."

The *principle* pertaining to that variety is this: When the health phenomenon at issue in an etiogenetic study is an event (rather than a state) and the etiogenesis at issue is not very acute – as was the case in all five of those studies – the proper comparative measure dictating the objects of study is rate ratio in the singular meaning of *incidence density* ratio (in a defined abstract domain); and the empirical counterpart of this from any study thus also properly is an IDR, this in reference to the population-time constituting the study base and the contrast of its index segment against its reference segment defined as of the person-moments constituting the study base (and not as of the persons' entries into the study base).

While the examples above were about diet – excessive in fats or deficient in antioxidants – in the etiogenesis of overt, symptomatic cancer, our added example is a related one and equally important: lack of 'screening' – really *lack of screening-associated presymptomatic treatments* – in the etiogenesis of *fatality from a cancer*.

Illustrative of the state of objects design in this research is a review of the results of this research in respect to breast cancer:

Demissie K et alii. Empirical comparison of the results of randomized trials and case-control studies in evaluating the effectiveness of screening mammography. *Journal of Clinical Epidemiology* 1998; 51: 81-91.

The idea was to derive "summary risk estimates" separately from each of the two types of study, for comparison in the spirit that, in principle, the same parameter was being quantified in each of the studies, even if the results of the two types of study may differ on account of incomplete adherence to the 'intervention' categories in the randomized trials.

The authors repeated the prevailing idea that "The gold standard for evaluating screening programs is the randomized controlled trial (RCT)" (sect. 2.6), adding that "Case-control studies are easier to perform but their role in this area is controversial." They gave several references to articles (and to one book) in which the principles of the 'case-control' studies on screening have been delineated.

Before getting to the particulars of that review, we give our introduction into the *principles* concerning the respective generic types of object that actually are addressed in those two types of study on the intended consequence of screening for a cancer.

That 'gold standard' RCT of epidemiological researchers and policy advocates regarding screening for a cancer is one in which seemingly healthy persons are randomly assigned to one of the two 'arms' of the trial. One of these commonly is simply that of 'usual care' (undefined, variable) in respect to the cancer, while in the other arm – the experimental one – of the study the care is defined to the extent that the participants are invited, or actually scheduled, to undergo periodic screenings for the cancer in terms of an initial test, with positive result of this test prompting referral to clinical care (for further diagnostics, undefined, and possible early treatment, undefined, upon rule-in diagnosis, undefined). The trial design involves specification of the time interval between successive rounds of the testing and also the number of these rounds, together with the duration of follow-up (as of randomization). The concern is to document the mortality from the cancer over the duration of the follow-up in each of the two arms of the trial – with a view to documentation of the proportional reduction in that mortality (due to the screening/testing).

The most eminent example of these 'gold standard' trials now is the most recent one, the National Lung Screening Trial in the U.S. Pertaining to it, the National Cancer Institute of the U.S. released, on 28 October 2010, a "statement" saying, among other things, that "The primary goal of the NLST was to determine whether [*sic*] three annual screenings with low-dose helical computerized tomography (LDCT) reduces mortality from lung cancer relative to screening with chest x-ray (CXR). The trial had been designed to have 90% statistical power for detecting 20% reduction in such mortality." The essential result prompting the trial's termination was that in the LDCT and CXR arms of the trial the respective rates of death from lung cancer over the 5–8 years of follow-up since entry into the trial were "245.7" and "308.3" per 100,000 person-years, and this was taken to imply a $(308.3 - 245.7)/308.3 = 20.3\%$ "reduction" in lung-cancer mortality by LDCT relative to CXR (Table 3 in the "statement"). The relative deficit in mortality from lung cancer in the LDCT arm "exceeded that expected by chance, even allowing for the multiple analyses conducted during the course of the trial," presumably taken to imply that the "reduction" was not due to chance.

Some editing is called for here. First, the mortality from lung cancer in the LDCT arm having been 20.3% lower than in the CXR arm does not mean that LDCT (really its associated treatments) reduced the mortality by 20.3% relative to what it would have been in the people in this arm of the trial had CXR been used instead of LCDT. And second, even though the trial was designed "for detecting 20% reduction in such mortality" (with 90% probability) and was stopped with the idea that the mission had been accomplished, in truth there was no such detection, nor could there have been. Reduction is an effect, and effect is not a phenomenon, subject to observation and, hence, detection and quantification (sect. 4.2). The reduction might have been 10%, or perhaps 40%; its specific magnitude is unknowable, that 20.3% being a composite of the reduction together with the workings of bias and chance. (The 95% 'confidence' interval, not given in the NCI "statement," is 6–31%.)

The "statistical power" calculation alluded to in that statement implies that associated with "three annual screenings with [LDCT]," instead of CXR, there is, if any, a particular degree of proportional reduction in mortality from lung cancer – a *constant* proportion over time as of the initiation of the screening, fully operative in whatever duration of follow-up.

Related to this is our *first principle* concerning the mortality reduction in a trial such as the NLST: The proportional reduction in mortality from the cancer is *nothing like a constant* over time from the beginning of the screening (for the generally short duration of it) to the end of the follow-up (for an arbitrary duration of it). It thus is logically inadmissible to quantify the reduction by pooling the experience across the entire duration of the follow-up. The proper concern in a trial like this is to address the incidence density of death from the cancer as a function of time since the initiation of the screening. And that function is, of course, different for different durations of the screening.

This leads to our related, *second principle*: Reduction in mortality from a cancer subsequent to screening can occur only if the cancer's treatments under the screening – those early treatments – are more commonly curative than those in the absence of screening. In fact, attainment of enhanced curability – by earlier treatments – is the very idea in screening for a cancer. Thus the parameter of Nature that should be viewed as the proper object of any study on the intended consequence of screening for a cancer is one that meaningfully quantifies the *gain in the cancer's curability rate* when screening-associated early treatments replace the treatments on already symptomatic cases in the absence of screening. This is a proportion of the cases of the cancer that are fatal in the absence of screening, the proportion of these otherwise fatal cases that are curable by screening-associated early treatments. Whatever may be the adopted design parameters for a trial such as the NLST in respect to the number of rounds of screening and the duration of follow-up, the proportional reduction in mortality as it is addressed in them (above) is prone to be much smaller than the curability gain just defined. But with sufficiently long-term screening, and focus on the appropriate segment of the follow-up, the magnitude of the curability gain can be studied in terms of a trial contrasting screening with no screening (ch. 11) – insofar as the necessary long-term adherence to the contrasted regimens can be effected.

This, in turn, leads to our *third principle*: A quantitatively meaningful etiogenetic study on death from a cancer, with lack of screening for it the etiogenetic factor, can be based on a case and base series from the relevant segment of follow-up in a screening trial with sufficiently long-term screening (and close adherence to the schedule). In the case series, the relevant history is about whether the person was under screening at the time of the cancer's detection (by virtue of being in the screening arm of the trial, irrespective of whether the diagnosis was derived on the prompting of a positive result of the initial test at issue or due to symptoms emerging between the scheduled tests). The corresponding histories in the base series involve some subtlety in respect to the corresponding times to which they refer, as set forth in section 11.5. The rate ratio (incidence-density ratio) from this study translates to (an empirical value for) the curability gain from early treatment.

With these principles as the background we now return to that review – 'meta-analysis' – by Demissie et alii (ref. above).

That report's Table 1 was entitled "Design, population and characteristics of screening approach of randomized control [*sic*] trials." As we noted above, critically important determinants of the magnitude of such mortality reduction as is addressed in these screening trials are the duration of the screening and the duration of the follow-up (as of randomization) – these, naturally, in addition to the nature of the entire regimen to pursue early diagnosis about the cancer, including the time interval between successive rounds of this regimen's application. That table reveals no specifics about the diagnostic regimens (not even their initial tests and the definitions of their positive results). The number of rounds of the screening is specified for each study (the range is from 1 to 7 among the trials), and specified also is the time interval between the rounds of screening (it was 12–33 months). It thus can be deduced that the durations of the screening ranged from 2 to 12 years. The duration of follow-up is specified, ranging from 7 to 16 years. Given the trials' great variability in such result-relevant aspects of their respective methodologies, no shared measure of mortality reduction – much less the practice-relevant parameter of Nature, the curability gain (regimen-specific) – was addressed as the object of study.

There thus was *no justification for deriving a single "summary risk estimate" from these "gold standard" studies*, trials that actually quantified a variety of highly arbitrary measures of mortality reduction – and with adherence to the screenings as low as 61% at one of the baseline rounds and 4% in one of the scheduled repeat rounds of screening. (Cf. sect. 2.6 re screening.)

The '*case-control*' studies (on lack of screening in the etiogenesis of death from breast cancer) had been conducted in settings into which routine availability of screening mammography had been introduced. Of particular note is the statement under Methods that "Exposure was defined as participation in one or more screening examinations from the beginning of the screening program up to the time of diagnosis of breast cancer in the case and the comparable time in the control." (Cf. "third principle" above).

Both trials (RCTs) and etiogenetic studies (non-experimental) on screening for a cancer need to address the *same parameter* of Nature characterizing the extent to which screening for a cancer has its intended consequence; they both need to quantify the gain in the cancer's curability afforded by screening-provided earlier detections of (earlier rule-in diagnoses about) the cancer – and the respective regimens of screening (pursuits of early diagnosis, and not merely the initial tests in it) as well as the treatments need to be both defined and 'comparable' (i.e., practically the same).

But: no meaningful quantity was addressed in any of the studies reviewed by Demissie et alii and, hence, in this review of those studies.

Principles of the study of the meaningfully construed intended consequence of screening for a cancer – the gain in the cancer's rate of curability – we address further in chapter 11.

7.3 The Result of the Design

Design of the objects of an etiologic/etiogenetic study – the parameters of Nature to be addressed in the study – is the result of designing an *occurrence relation* for the outcome phenomenon together with the domain for this (sect. 4.4). For, the study's object parameters are imbedded in this adopted model, generally along with some 'nuisance parameters' having to do with making the outcome's occurrence in relation to the etiogenetic determinant suitably conditional to imply (as best can be judged) that relation's causal nature (sect. 4.4).

It deserves emphasis that this model, while medical in its substance, is *statistical* in form. Medically one thinks about the outcome's rate of occurrence in the domain, and specifically about the way in which this rate depends, causally, on the history in respect to the (potentially) etiogenetic factor at issue; and the rate-ratio's modifiers along with potential confounders of the causal relation also enter into this medical thinking. In the designed occurrence relation, the outcome's rate of occurrence is represented by a chosen *occurrence measure*, ordinarily the logarithm of the numerical element in the outcome event's incidence density (sect. 4.4). The magnitude of this measure is formulated as a function (linear) of a set of *statistical variates* (numerical) adopted ad hoc as representations of the person characterizers on which this magnitude depends – according to the design of the occurrence relation that defines the objects – the *object parameters* – of the study.

We emphasize this because it represents a major departure from the prevailing thinking and practice in etiogenetic research. As it is, quite sharp a distinction is being made between '*study design*' and the study's '*data analysis,*' so that the study design does not define the parameters – the objects of study – the empirical values of which are to be derived by suitable synthesis (*sic*) of the data – by suitable fitting of (the operational counterpart of) the designed occurrence relation to the data. We thus emphasize the *need to integrate* the medical and statistical aspects of the research – just as the material and mathematical aspects are integrated in physics (in, e.g., Maxwell's equations on electromagnetic radiation).

We thus emphasize the need to think of etiogenetic research as inquiry into the magnitudes of defined *statistical parameters of Nature*, whether qualitatively (as to existence of deviations from their null values) or quantitatively (as to the magnitudes of those deviations).

7.4   Implications of the Design

The here strongly advocated explicit, up-front design of the objects of study, and this, specifically, as a matter of design all the way to the *statistical form* of the occurrence relation implying the statistical objects of (the statistical parameters for) study, has as its most straightforward implication the conceptual *form of the result* – that the result is empirical rate-ratio as a function of certain modifiers of its magnitude, as we already have noted.

A related, minor implication is that an etiogenetic study's objects design implicitly defines the *objective* of the study: to produce *evidence* about the magnitudes of the parameters that were designed to constitute the objects of the study.

Very important is the objects design's bearing on the study's *methods design*. Suffice it here to refer back to sections 2.2 and 7.2 and, for example, the discussions there of how seriously misleading has been all of the research – purportedly critically relevant randomized trials included – on diets deficient in their antioxidant content in the etiogenesis of cancers. Without due regard for deliberate and thoughtful – and also knowledge-driven – objects design, these trials' methodologic routines have implied results in reference to very recent diets (or diet supplementations) on the scale of etiogenetic time (retrospective as of the time of the occurrence/non-occurrence of the cancer's entering the 'clinical' phase of its development). Proper attention to objects design, we argued, would call for the causal contrast to refer to the earliest decades of life, with the domain for the outcome's occurrence representing rather late decades of life. And we noted, too, that insofar as the nature of a meaningfully designed set of objects makes the study methodologically impracticable, refraining from study is preferable to a study that is inherently misleading on account of the form of its result.

Finally, what has here been said about objects design for etiogenetic studies implies the need to stop classifying etiogenetic researchers as being either *'epidemiologists'* or *'biostatisticians,'* as this fosters disintegration of the medical and statistical aspects of the research, while integration of these two really is called for (cf. above). And once the necessary integration takes manifestation in the objects design in terms of an occurrence relation with statistical variates and statistical parameters, Statistical Methods vanishes from the study report while Objects Design enters.

Chapter 8
Etiologic Studies' Methods Design

Abstract Once the study's objects design has defined what the investigators are concerned to shed light on – the values of what parameters of Nature in what domain, conditionally on what extraneous determinants on the outcome phenomenon's rate of occurrence – they can turn their attention to the study's *methods design*. In it they define how they aim to 'measure' those parameters' values – ultimately by means of fitting the logistic counterpart of the objects-defining log-linear model for the outcome's occurrence to the data (the realizations of Y, X_1, X_2, ...) on the study's case and base series. The resulting empirical rate-ratio function translates into the result for the etiogenetic proportion of interest (chap. 4 Abstract).

The methods design of an etiogenetic study proceeds in two distinct stages. In the first stage, the objects-defining occurrence relation that was designed in reference to Nature in the abstract is adapted to the actual study, translated into the *operationalized model*. The independent variates in the logistic model to be fitted are defined in reference to this counterpart of the theoretical model. The second stage of the methods design defines the means by which *empirical content* of that form is judged to be best obtained. While the essence of the study has an a-priori definition, many particulars of it remain to be specified/designed (chap. 6 Abstract).

This second stage of the study's methods design is governed by the imperative of *validity* assurance, descriptively, together with the desideratum of *efficiency* optimization. Both of these, in turn, are governed by principles of the studies' methods design.

Apart from efficiency, a determinant of the study's *informativeness* is its size; but this is not subject to principles-guided optimization, with one exception: when a violation of principle is detected in the study's objects design or in its methods design in respects other than study size (number of datapoints in the two series), the optimal – indeed, correct – size of the study is zero.

8.1   Some Considerations in the Design

The methods design of an etiologic/etiogenetic study should be understood to be constrained by the *methodologic implications of the objects design* for the study. After all, the study's methodology is the means to the study's preset end – the objective of attaining (new) evidence about the magnitudes of the study's object parameters. And another overarching constraint, just as critical, is the need to appreciate the *singular essence* of the study (sect. 6.5), even though this leaves for consideration the menu of design topics and their corresponding *design options* (sect. 6.6).

For the actual study, the elements in the designed occurrence relation need to be given their respective *operational definitions*. For example, while the study domain (abstract) generally is one of no previous occurrence of the outcome at issue, the operational criteria for this need to be defined. And, as another example, when the outcome at issue (as is typical) is the event of the illness making, in its progression, the transition from a latent, preclinical stage to the overt, clinical stage, the operational counterpart of this needs to be defined.

The statistical variates (Xs) in the designed occurrence relation are defined in reference to various person characterizers in the abstract; but those variates need to be replaced by their operational counterparts, ones in reference to the operational counterparts of the conceptual determinants of the outcome's (rate of) occurrence (in the abstract domain). For example and most notably, definition is needed for the way the histories on the etiogenetic determinant are to be ascertained, preparatory to these ascertainments and their translations into realizations of the corresponding variates in the definition of the objects of study.

All of these considerations, and other similar ones also, are directly related to the designed occurrence relation, including the potential confounders in it. But they indeed are ones of the study's methodology and not ones of reformulation of the objects of the study. One does not, in this research, study the operational, but one necessarily is operational in studying the non-operational, the abstract. The beginning of this, in etiogenetic research, is that something noumenal (causation) is being studied in terms of matters phenomenal (sect. 4.2) – empirical.

In the rest of the methodology, the first set of considerations generally relates to the *source population*; and in this, the very first component consideration generally should be whether it can be simply selected/defined, or whether, instead, it needs to be operationally formed. For, a usable source population is one in which sufficiently well-ascertainable histories in relevant respects – most notably as to the etiogenetic determinant at issue – are associated with each person-moment in it; and it can be, as in the Framingham Heart Study and the Nurses' Health Study, that facts on the source population (a cohort in each of these examples) need to be prospectively 'observed' and documented to make the histories for the case and base series of subsequent etiogenetic studies ascertainable and, hence, documentable.

If this preparatory facts-recording (burdensome, time-consuming) is deemed not to be needed, then the highest-priority considerations generally have to do with the way in which the source population will be selected/defined. The chosen definition may be direct; or it may be indirect, as the catchment population secondary to the way in which cases of the outcome are identified (to which direct definition is given).

Either way, an important methodological consideration is the operational definition of the *illness at issue*, notably as to whether it should be restricted to cases are in their manifestations typical and also severe – for reasons of helping to assure validity of the study. This restriction in the operational definition of a case of the illness facilitates complete case identification from a directly defined source population; and it makes more concrete the source population with indirect definition of it, thereby facilitating its fair sampling of the source base (for the first-stage base series; sect. 5.2).

Among the orientational considerations also is this: Should the conditionality of the outcome's rate of occurrence on potential confounders, called for by the study's objects design, indeed be pursued in terms of documentation and control, or should this be replaced by *prevention of the confounding* – by redesign of the occurrence relation or suitable design of the study base as representation of the domain? For example, as smoking represents a generally poorly controllable potential confounder, the solution may be restriction of study domain to life-long non-smokers. As another example, confounding by the level of fever in the study of aspirin use in the etiogenesis of Reye's syndrome in the domain of febrile illness in childhood may be prevented by contrasting aspirin use with the use of another antipyretic (acetaminophen, say). On the other hand, prevention of confounding by socio-economic status in the study of etiogenesis by occupational exposure to a toxin may be accomplished by forming the source population of workers in such a way that the exposure at issue can be presumed to be, in this population, uncorrelated with SES (cf. sect. 6.4). In experimental causal research, the preeminent means of prevention of confounding, specific to T_0 of cohort and scientific time, is randomization, while prospective confounding may be prevented by blinding (which may require placebo comparison).

These examples might suffice to convey the point that even though 'cohort,' 'case-control,' and 'cross-sectional' study do not represent defensible design alternatives to each other in etiogenetic research (sect. 6.5), there really are options – very notable ones – in the study's methods design beyond the operational reformulation of the objects-defining occurrence relation together with its domain (sect. 6.6).

8.2   Some Principles of the Design

The overarching principle in an etiologic/etiogenetic study's methods design – in the operationalization of the designed occurrence relation and in the design of the study proper – is the imperative to assure a reasonable degree of *validity* for the study, complete validity generally being unattainable. Another, secondary concern – desideratum rather than an imperative – is maximization of the study's *efficiency*, within the limits of the attainable.

An etiogenetic study's validity can be, and needs to be, thought of in two stages. The study is *descriptively* valid to the extent that the object parameters' empirical values in its result would converge to those of the corresponding parameters of Nature (defined by the designed occurrence relation) were the study size to approach infinity (so that chance imprecision of the empirical values would be fully eliminated). Insofar as those parameters have 'locally' (in the study's place and at its time) specific values, then this amounts to definition of the study's local validity, in descriptive terms. And the study is *causally* (etiogenetically) valid to the extent that its result is not only descriptively valid but also free of confounding.

Lack of validity in an etiogenetic study is, most broadly, of one or more of three types. It is constituted by selection bias and/or documentation bias taking away from descriptive validity and, of course, by confounding bias as a potential added element in the lack of causal validity.

Selection bias results from violation of one or both of two principles. One of these principles is that commitment to the source base must be made independently of even a hunch about what the result from the study base in it, specifically, would be; and by the same token, the commitment must be adhered to independently of the findings from what was designed to be the study base. The associated other principle is that a study base (within the source base) must be the result of the study subjects' entries into and exits from it independently of the outcome itself. This generally means entries and exits independently of precursors (prodromata) of the outcome. However, for validity of etiogenetic study, actually required is only that there not be differential dependence on precursors of the outcome between the contrasted experiences.

Selection bias of that first kind is akin to result-dependent submission of the study report for publication, and to the study report's result-dependent acceptance for publication. Both of these violations of principle – very common and knowingly committed! – conduce to 'publication bias' in the aggregate of published studies on any given (set of) object(s) of study, and this in turn makes for unavoidable selection bias in the study base of any derivative study on the magnitudes of the object parameter(s) (sect. 13.1). Publication bias could be eliminated by a simple innovation in medical journalism (sect. 13.6).

Selection bias of that second kind is tantamount to the study base being distorted by failures in the implementation of the protocol. By the same token, its prevention is a matter of stringent adherence to the protocol in its implementation, so long as the protocol itself is sound.

Documentation bias, in sharp contrast to selection bias, is not at all about the study base per se. Whatever the study base is, the occurrence relation in it – the operationalized counterpart of what was designed in reference to the abstract – should be documented correctly, validly in this sense. In this documentation, bias is a consequence of contravention of one or more of the three principles of it: the production the two series (case and base series) must be valid for their shared referent, the study base; these two series must be correctly documented in respect to the person-characteristics represented by the realizations of the statistical variates in the operationalized version of the designed occurrence relation; and the study objects' operationalized version must accord with the theoretical one.

With secondary definition of the source population (as the cases' catchment population), the case series inherently is complete for the source base and, hence, for the study base, but valid sampling of the indirectly defined source population (at whatever time) is a major challenge; and when the source population is defined directly, there generally is a sampling frame for its valid sampling, but complete (and valid incomplete) identification the cases occurring in the source base poses a major challenge.

When direct definition is given to how the cases are identified, a first step in making the catchment population more concrete (for more valid sampling of it) can be basing it on canvassing all of the care facilities in which the cases are diagnosed within a contiguous, large region (a metropolitan area, say) and restricting the cases' admissibility (and thereby the study base) to residents of that region.

More to the same effect is changing the operational definition of case to one that is severe and clinically typical. For if the case is severe, the person is more likely to seek medical attention; and if it is clinically – in its symptoms and signs – typical, its recognition for what it is, is more likely.

With these arrangements for the development of the case series for an etiogenetic study, the source base becomes quite concrete in its definition; in fact, it gets to be indistinguishable from one in the context of the source population having been given of the primary, direct definition. And if the source population is defined directly, its associated challenge of valid case identification would be more manageable by pursuing it in the manner just outlined for it in the context of the source population's secondary, indirect definition. With these arrangements the otherwise major duality constituted by the two ways of defining the source population becomes moot.

Even though a concrete definition of the source population generally provides for statistical sampling of the source population/base, it may be preferable, for validity assurance, to sample it by the use of *extraneous outcome* events, to help assure that the reported histories in the base series are of the same accuracy as in the case and base series. Valid outcomes for this purpose are ones whose occurrence is uninfluenced by the etiogenetic determinant at issue.

When sampling the base by suitable extraneous outcome events, two important questions relate to this: How many types of such an outcome? and, How identified? We hold that a good number generally is three, as a number larger than one allows checking their postulated interchangeability under the premise that each of them is suitable, while an unduly large number has two drawbacks: it takes away from the informativeness in these interchangeability assessments, and it imposes undue burdens to colleagues in their judgements about the tenability of the premise that each of the events is suitable for the purpose.

The identification of the extraneous outcome events for the base series – generally all of them, as defined, occurring in the study base – is to be, in relevant respects, completely analogous to that for the case series: definition of the admissible cases, canvassing all of the care facilities for them (*sic*), etc. (see above). This makes (the common practice of) matching by hospital inadmissible whenever the care facilities for the extraneous cases differ from those for the cases of interest.

The distribution of the case series (by a correlate of the etiogenetic history) can be used as a (partial) guide for stratification of the sampling for the base series, the other guides being the histories' varied distributions and the sampling's varied unit costs across the strata. (See efficiency below.)

If the base sampling is stratified by person-characterizers other than what already is involved in the designed (and operationalized) occurrence relation, the stratification factors need to be added to those in the pre-designed occurrence relation (i.e., the result is to be made conditional on these, too).

Confounding bias in the result of an etiogenetic study has two possible sources: the designed theoretical occurrence relation may (and commonly does) fail to make the objects of study sufficiently conditional on extraneous determinants of the outcome's (rate of) occurrence; and the operationalized counterpart of this conditioning may be deficient as a representation of that conditioning.

Insufficient conditionality on extraneous determinants in the theoretical occurrence relation is not inherently a matter of the set of accounted-for potential confounders being incomplete. Another source of the problem is inadequate conceptualization – and hence inadequate representation – of a determinant that is accounted for. For example, history of smoking likely is, generally, quite inadequately accounted for by inclusion, in the log-linear model, of a single term for pack-years of cigarette smoking. The same is true of a single term for years of education in conditioning for socio-economic status. And when use of aspirin has been studied in the etiology of Reye's syndrome in the domain of febrile illness in childhood, a major concern has been potential confounding by the level of the fever, the meaning of which is obfuscated by the antipyretic effect of the aspirin use.

When problems in the conceptualization and/or documentation of a confounder (or in the modeling of its role as a determinant) are unsurmountable, making *control* of confounding (characterizing the study base) impracticable, the need is to consider possible attainability of *prevention* of confounding (from characterizing the study base); see section 8.1 above.

Efficiency optimization, like validity assurance, for an etiogenetic study begins in the study's objects design, as for the *domain* in the occurrence relation. For a start, the domain must satisfy the most elementary requirements for the study objects' (parameters') studyability: the domain must be one in which the outcome of interest occurs; and it must also be one in which the determinant of interest varies. Thus, when studying the occurrence of deep-vein thrombosis (or its consequent pulmonary embolism) in causal relation to recent use of an oral contraceptive, both of these elementary requirements are satisfied only by women of childbearing age. Study in a domain that does not satisfy these simply qualitative requirements would be extremely inefficient. Its information yield in relation to its cost (monetary and other) would be extremely low, as its informativeness would be nil.

The efficiency-optimal *rate of occurrence* of the outcome (in the domain of the study) is a topic of some subtlety. If the cost of assembling (and documenting) a given number of cases of the outcome is the same in a lower-rate domain as in a higher-rate one, more efficient for hypothesis-testing is prone to be a study in the lower-rate domain, given also that the distribution of the contrasted histories on the determinant of concern is the same in these two domains. For where other causes are less common, the rate-ratio for the cause at issue tends to be more pronounced in its deviation from unity (as this cause is a more salient one in the relative absence of others).

To wit, the role of in-utero exposure to mother's use of DES (diethyl stilbestrol, to sustain pregnancy) in the etiogenesis of clear-cell carcinoma of the vagina was evident from a mere one dozen cases of this disease because this exposure is a quite unique cause of this very rare disease. If the disease were much more common, it would have a high etiogenetic proportion for causes other than in-utero exposure to DES; the proportion of the cases with this DES antecedent would be much lower; the factor-conditional etiogenetic proportion for this DES exposure would be much lower; and the rate-ratio pertaining to it would be much closer to unity. A dozen cases of the disease would, thus, be much less informative about the existence of the DES etiogenesis (when considered in conjunction with a suitable base series).

As for the contrasted *histories' variability* in the study domain, the efficiency-optimal distribution naturally is that of maximal variability – near-equal frequencies for the index and reference histories (with no 'other' histories). Thus, a particular choice of the domain is efficiency-enhancing if it means greater variability of the etiogenetic histories, *ceteris paribus*.

The variability of the contrasted etiogenetic histories is subject to methodologic enhancement as well. In particular, when a cohort is formed to serve as the source population, the histories' variability in the prospective study base should not be determined solely by this cohort's source population (generally dynamic). Instead, it should be enhanced by means of selective enrollments into the cohort with a view to efficient variability of the histories at cohort T_0, aiming at either the 'two-point design' (accenting, equally, the histories' extremes) or the 'three-point design' (with a third group in the middle).

In contravention of this principle, very notably, the cohort for the ever-so-eminent Framingham Heart Study was selected as a representative sample of the targeted segment of the town's population, the consequence being the very opposite of what would have been efficient: accented got to be the middle instead of the extremes. (Nature has no propensity to optimize the efficiency of epidemiological studies: it is left for the investigators to pursue.)

When the decision has been taken to conduct an etiogenetic study in a given setting, there commonly is an opportunity to enhance the study's informativeness (its result's precision) by increasing the size of the case series (by increasing the size of the study base) and/or by increasing the size of the base series. This raises the question about the efficiency-optimal relative sizes of these two series when both of them can be expanded; and the answer is that optimal is the size ratio that is the inverse of the square root of the unit-cost ratio between the two series. But if the size of the case series is a given, the study's informativeness can be increased only by increasing the size of the base series – which does not provide appreciable further increase once the base series already is, say, fivefold in size relative to the case series. A large base series is prone to be cost-ineffective, inefficient.

Among the distributional determinants of an etiogenetic study's efficiency also is the designed distribution of the base series across strata of the study base. It remains commonplace to match the base series to the case series, meaning that it is chosen so as to have identical distributions for the two series, by gender and age, for example; but this is not efficiency-optimal (while irrelevant for validity). Efficiency-optimal is sampling that is proportional to informativeness and inversely proportional to the square root of unit-cost of the sampling; and a stratum's informativeness is proportional not only to the number of cases from it but also to the product of the proportional sizes of the index and reference segments of the stratum-specific segments of the study base.

8.3   Implications of the Design

Once the objects design for an etiologic/etiogenetic study has been followed by its corresponding methods design, the investigators are ready to produce the *study protocol*, which defines, in all relevant detail, the study methodology – all the way to the synthesis of the collected data into the study result together with its associated measures of the imprecisions of the empirical values of the object parameters.

The study protocol has direct bearing on the study report, the core of which is *evidence* about the object parameters in dual terms: the study *result* together with its associated measures of imprecision for one, and the *genesis* of these numerics for another – with description of the salient features of the protocol the core input to the latter, supplemented by information about deviations from it in the implementation of the designed methodology.

The study protocol commonly is to be supplemented by the study's *manual of operations* or, as a modern counterpart of this, a *web-based management system*, governing and guiding the study procedures with a view to quality assurance in respect to adherence to the protocol.

Insofar as the operationalized version of the occurrence relation is true to the theoretical one it represents and the rest of the methodology indeed is, as intended, practicable and successfully implemented, the ultimate implication of this is that the study result will be, in essence, descriptively unbiased (sect. 8.2 above). The extent to which a descriptively unbiased result also is causally unbiased is a question of the study's methodology; but it also is a question of its objects design (sect. 8.2 above).

The study result's degree of causal unbiasedness together with its precision determine the *burden of evidence* from the study. The precision is determined by the study's efficiency together with its *size*.

It bears emphasis that there are not, nor can there be, tenable principles of *optimizing the size* of an etiogenetic study – the number of datapoints (person-moments) in its study (case and base) series – save for one: for a study with an identifiable violation of tenable principles in its objects design or methods design, the optimal size is zero. Any scheme of 'sample-size determination' is but a mapping of an arbitrarily selected value for a measure of the result's precision to its corresponding size of the study; and the result derived from it is commonly changed, drastically, by reviewers of the grant application – to zero (with corresponding adjustment of the budget).

Chapter 9
Etiologic Studies' Intervention Counterparts

Abstract In regard to population-level epidemiological research, the concern in this text has thus far been with the overwhelmingly most common genre of this, namely, causal research of the etiogenetic rather than interventive genre (chap. 3 Abstract); but the causal research can also be of the latter type, notably in studying the health effects of *preventive interventions* – vaccinations, for example.

While etiogenetic research generally is about unintended effects, current, of matters in people's past (constitutional, environmental, behavioral), interventive research is mainly about *intended effects*, prospective, of actions (interventive) taken prospectively, with the aim of changing the future course of health for the better. It thus is, mainly, about *effectiveness* of interventions.

Intervention being a purposive action, with a defined alternative (possibly inaction), it is subject to *experimental* study, in which the choice of intervention is governed by the concern to learn about alternative interventions' relative effects – rather than to achieve an intervention's known (or presumed) effect.

In an intervention study, even if only quasi-experimental, the *objects of study* have to do with a domain of indications (and absence of contraindications) for the contrasted interventions. They are imbedded in a designed occurrence relation for prospective intervention-time, with the determinant of interest characterized by prospective divergence between the contrasted interventions, defined as algorithms of intervention throughout the designed time horizon for the outcome's occurrence.

An intervention study, like an etiogenetic study, should lead to a *case series and a base series* from the study base, which here is the study cohort's population-time of follow-up. And in particular, the base series should be a simple, representative (rather than stratified) sample of the study base. For this allows the resulting rate-ratio function to be translated into its corresponding incidence-density function, which in turn can be translated into the corresponding *prognostic probability function* for the outcome of interventive concern.

Experimental intervention research raises particular *ethical* issues, which remain incompletely understood and poorly dealt with.

O.S. Miettinen and I. Karp, *Epidemiological Research: An Introduction*,
DOI 10.1007/978-94-007-4537-7_9, © Springer Science+Business Media Dordrecht 2012

9.1   The Eminence of Experiments

Etiologic/etiogenetic research generally is non-experimental (ch. 6), meaning that the causal determinant's histories in the study base are not artificially – experimentally – arranged for the purposes of the study; the history associated with any given person- moment in the study base got to be what it is quite independently of the study. The particular reasons for the non-experimental nature of etiogenetic studies, not shared by their intervention counterparts, are scientific-practical for one and ethical for another.

An experimental study base in etiogenetic research would commonly need to be deeply prospective in study time. For, from the vantage of the person-moments in the study base, the experimentally arranged etiogenetic histories would commonly need to be quite longitudinal, and this requires at least equally longitudinal prospective work in an experimental etiogenetic study. Apart from the tedium, a major problem is that long-term adherence to the experimental regimen, whatever it is, would commonly be unattainable.

The ethical obstacle to experimental research on etiogenesis generally is the qualitative nature of the causal contrast: even in hypothesis-testing there generally cannot be experts' equipoise between the merits of a person being assigned to one of the determinant's index categories versus the reference category of it – the former typically representing a (prospective) health hazards without countervailing benefit, potentially at least, while the hazards would assuredly be absent in the determinant's reference category. Even if there were properly informed volunteers for participation in such a study, solicitation of their participation is generally regarded as ethically inadmissible (sect. 9.4).

These prohibitive ethical considerations do not apply to hypothesis-testing about (potential) etiogenesis by quantitatively suboptimal but unknown levels of something that generally is (or at least is presumed) to be needed for maintenance of good health – things such as fluorine in one's drinking-water environment (sect. 4.1) and antioxidant intake as a matter of one's behavior in respect to diet and dietary supplements (sect. 2.2).

In contrast to etiogenetic research, epidemiological *intervention* research generally is experimental even on the population level (and not only on the 'bench' level). One practically enabling factor is that experimental intervention is no more of an artifact than is intervention in actual practice of healthcare (preventive). Even the general ethical obstacle to experimental etiogenetic research on humans (above) is absent from truly pragmatic intervention research as experts' equipoise is inherent in the contrast, which is between/among candidates for the intervention of choice. And whereas the outcome phenomena generally are prospective in study time, so inherently also are the interventions (different from causal histories in etiogenetic studies).

Finally, experimentation in the particular meaning of a randomized contrast may actually be needed. It may be needed for prevention of confounding by indication, which is a topic peculiar to the intentional causation by intervention, distinct from the generally unintentional causation in the etiogenesis of illnesses as they naturally occur, and which tends not to lend itself to documentation and control based on this. Another, obvious, need for experimentation – and it can just as well randomized – attends to the situation in which at least one of the contending interventions of choice is not (yet) in routine use.

9.2 The Objects of the Studies

In *etiologic*/etiogenetic studies, quite generally, the histories pertaining to a given contrast can readily be supplemented by other, unrelated contrasts. Thus, a contrast which in itself justifies an etiogenetic study generally justifies addressing some *ancillary contrasts*, their study by means of the same case and base series: several substantively distinct studies can be efficiently conflated into what procedurally is, in essence, a single study.

In *intervention* studies of the usual, '*parallel*' type, the counterpart of etiogenetic studies' necessary case series together with its corresponding base series is their necessary study cohort together with the intervention contrast in it, prospective, as of cohort T_0. And while intervention studies generally are justified by inquiry into the compared interventions' relative effectiveness in producing the intended effect, this is readily supplemented by consideration of other, *ancillary outcomes*, generally ones that have to do with the interventions' (potential) unintended effects. Again, several substantively distinct studies can be conflated into what procedurally is, in essence, a single study. We discuss the alternative to these parallel trials – the 'before-after' trials, that is – at the end of section 9.3 below.

The objects of any population-level epidemiological study are defined, as we have set forth, by a designed occurrence relation – a health phenomenon's rate of occurrence as a function of determinants of this rate, in a particular domain of this occurrence. We have not, however, emphasized that both the domain and the occurrence relation in it are defined on the scale of *scientific time*, which in turn is defined by its inherent zero point, T_0. This scale of time is distinct from such particularistic scales of time as study time (T_0: the time of the inception of data collection) and cohort time (T_0: the time of entry into the cohort).

While in the study base of any etiogenetic study the scientific time at each of its person-moments is the time of the outcome and, thus, $T = T_0$ in etiogenetic time (retrospective, $T < T_0 = 0$), in any interventive study the scientific time is some $T > T_0$ in intervention-prognostic time at each of the person-moments in its study base, T_0 being the time as of which the intervention status diverges (this being the time, also, of cohort T_0 for the study population). In each of these two types of study, a person-moment in the domain of the object of study is one of occurrence/non-occurrence of the outcome phenomenon in question.

While the *object* of any given etiogenetic study is the outcome phenomenon's rate of occurrence at T_0 of etiogenetic time, this in causal relation to retrospective, pre-T_0 divergence in the causal determinant, that of any given interventive study is the outcome phenomenon's prospective, post-T_0 rate of occurrence on the scale of intervention time, this in causal relation to prospective, post-T_0 divergence in the causal determinant.

In etiogenetic studies the designed *temporal relation* between the outcome's occurrence and its causal determinant is, in principle at least, dictated by Nature – the histories need to cover, in principle, the entire range of time (retrospective) in which the factor can have exerted its etiogenetic effect. If the object of study is designed to focus on a limited segment of the full range of etiogenetic time, then histories in respect to the other segments represent potential confounders. But in interventive studies, by contrast, the corresponding temporal relation is dictated, in its entirety, by the investigators. The investigators commonly opt for studying the outcome's (rate of) occurrence in a limited, early segment (prospective) of the scientific time, occurrence in this period in causal relation to the causal (interventive) determinant of this as of the scientific T_0 – with the outcome's timing quite possibly an element in the designed occurrence relation and with no role for the later ranges of prospective time; the object function is understood to pertain only to a limited range of prospective time.

Another difference relates to this. In an etiogenetic study, concerning a given (potentially) etiogenetic factor, there may be concern to distinguish among various periods of etiogenetic time – 'recent,' 'intermediate,' and 'distant' past, say, each expressly defined – leading to their corresponding, separate etiogenetic determinants for joint inclusion in the designed occurrence relation. In an interventive study there generally is a counterpart of this but there is no imperative to address the entire range of the relevant prognostic time: in particular, no confounding arises from whatever may be happening in the segment of time that is not addressed.

9.3   The Methods in the Experiments

The *source population* in an intervention experiment, very different from its counterpart in non-experimental etiologic/etiogenetic studies, is, in a segment of its *prospective* course in study time, a source for identification of *candidates for enrollment* into the study population, inherently the *study cohort*. These are persons who, at the time of the identification, are seen to apparently represent presence of the (designed) indication for the intervention(s) and freedom from the (designed) contra-indications for it/them, while also apparently satisfying whatever other (designed) criteria of admissibility into the study cohort. (Those admissibility criteria are defined by the operationalized version of the initially designed occurrence relation; cf. sect. 8.1.) The source population can be, for example, a segment of the listeners of a set of radio stations.

Given an identified case (person-moment) of apparent eligibility for enrollment into the study cohort, the investigators may – but need not – proceed to *solicitation* of the person's potential volunteering to the enrollment, following whatever non-scientific preliminaries to this (sect. 9.4 below). If the consent to (potential) enrollment is sought and obtained, this may initially be followed only by tentative enrollment. For, the admissibility criteria may need to be assessed more comprehensively and/or more closely; and there may be a need to furtively test the person's adherence to an agreed-upon plan for some simulated intervention.

The process leading to a person's definite *enrollment* into the study cohort is completed if, and when, the assignment – experimental, generally randomization-based – to a particular intervention occurs. This is the study cohort's membership-clinching event, after which there will be no exit from the membership (sect. 6.1). This study population is formed from, rather than embedded in, the source population (cf. sect. 5.1), and it thus has its (prospective) course independently from that of its source population (which usually is open – dynamic – rather than closed).

Two tasks are executed at the time of a person's enrollment into the study cohort, at this T_0 of cohort time as well as of actual scientific time. One of these tasks naturally is *documentation* of the relevant facts which, in the operationalized (methodological) version of the initially designed occurrence relation, have this T_0 as their temporal referent. And the other one, just as naturally, is the *assignment of the intervention*, possibly with *blinding* of the assignment (for prevention of prospective confounding and/or assurance of validity of outcome assessment). If one of the 'interventions' actually is no intervention at all, it may need to be represented by *placebo* intervention in the context of blinding.

In the post-T_0 period, too, there are two tasks to be executed. One of these again is a matter of observation and it related *documentation*, while the other one is in the nature of *execution* and *enforcement*, having to do with the commitments of the study subjects and, notably, those of the research personnel too. The documentation has to do with protocol adherence for one, and with the outcomes – both effectiveness- and safety-related – for another. And the execution and enforcement of the intervention commitment is a post-T_0 task even in the context of an acute intervention, given that the protocol specifies this as the only (*sic*) intervention (so long as the documented outcomes may be affected by extraneous interventions).

Given that all that is to be performed in the post-T_0 (post-randomization) period in an intervention experiment, 'follow-up' is too passive-sounding as a term for it. To wit, studied are *effects of actual interventions*, not those of intentions to be subjected to an intervention (or to its defined alternative; sect. 3.1). Effects in medicine, and in its simulated practice in intervention experiments likewise, characterize actions, not mere intentions to act; and they can be unintended as well as intended effects of actions, never of mere intentions to act.

Once the data have been collected and entered into the trial's database, the outcome events of a given type (those relevant of effectiveness, say) that occurred in the study base can be identified from the database, and as a supplement to this *case series* can be selected a suitable *base series* – as in a logically construed etiogenetic study (sect. 6.5). For each of these two series, the database allows the identification of the type of the intervention and the duration of this (since T_0); and the same is true of all other relevant information (incl. that documented at T_0).

Fitting the logistic counterpart of the designed log-linear model for the outcome event's incidence density to the data (the designed statistical variates' realizations) in the two series, results in a documentation of the experience in terms of the event's incidence-density ratio as a function of intervention time (T), type of intervention, and the person's prognostic indicator profile at T_0.

But as at issue actually is not an etiogenetic study but an interventive one, the interest is not in the (causal) rate ratio but the *rate proper*, the event's *incidence density* as a joint function of all of those determinants of its level. To derive this function for the incidence density of the outcome event at issue, a *representative* (simple random) sample of the study base is to be drawn to constitute the base series. Then, the desired function for incidence density can be derived as

$$ID = (B/PT) \exp(L),$$

where B is the size of the base series, PT is the amount of population time constituting the study base, and L is the linear compound arising from the logistic model's fitting to the data on the case and base series. The corresponding empirical function for cumulative incidence and *risk* from time $T = 0$ to $T = t$ is

$$CI_{0,t} = 1 - \exp\left(-\int_0^t ID_t dt\right).$$

When the outcome at issue is a *state* of health and the concern thus is to derive the corresponding *prevalence* function, the base series need not be derived by representative sampling; the only requirement is that it be independent of the presence/absence of the outcome state at the sampled person-moment. For, the designed prevalence function is fitted to this single series, with no involvement of quasi-rates and rate ratio. The logistic model for the prevalence is fitted to the data. The logit of the prevalence at $T = t$, in the study base, is taken to be the resulting function's realization at this point in time since the interventive T_0.

In an intervention trial of that usual, *parallel* type, any intervention contrast is an asymmetrical one, just as is any etiogenetic contrast. The concern is not to compare one intervention with another one. Instead, the concern is with only one intervention at a time, with its effect on the (rate of) occurrence of the outcome at issue when this intervention – the *index* intervention in the contrast – is present in lieu of its defined alternative – the *reference* intervention – in the contrast. The role of the reference 'arm' in the trial is to provide for surmising what the outcome's rate of occurrence in the index arm would have been had this subcohort been subjected to the reference intervention instead of the index intervention (cf. sect. 4.3).

This parallel arrangement is needed when, as is usual, one of these two conditions obtains: the alternative indeed is an actual intervention, another possible intervention of choice; or it is absence of any actual intervention but the outcome's rate of occurrence in the absence of any intervention cannot be presumed to be (practically) constant over the follow-up time in the trial.

By the same token, there is no need for a reference arm when an intervention is contrasted with no intervention and the outcome's rate of occurrence can be presumed to be (practically) constant over a period of time before and after the initiation of the intervention, given no effect of the intervention. In this situation, a *before-after* trial will do: the change in the outcome's (rate of) occurrence from before the intervention to what it is after (the initiation of) the intervention is a measure of the intervention's effect as such (being that practically no change can be presumed to occur in the absence of the intervention).

9.4   The Ethics in the Experiments

In population-level epidemiological research, the issues in the studies' objects design and methods design correspond to *ontology* and *epistemology* in philosophy, the mother of all of science. For, in ontology philosophers contemplate what is 'real' and hence possibly worth knowing about, while in epistemology they contemplate how knowledge about a 'real' thing (entity, quality/quantity, or relation) could be gained.

Ontology and epistemology are quite unrelated to a third eminent branch of philosophy, to 'moral philosophy' or *ethics*. In this the concern is to understand what is morally good or bad, right or wrong, in human *action*, as it has to do with other creatures, *humans* in particular. Population-level epidemiological research is human action, of course; and it has to do with other humans, in two fundamental ways: it seeks knowledge (scientific) for the benefit of humans at large, and to this end it can involve imposition of something undesirable on some humans. Philosophy of ethics therefore has direct bearing on research on humans, on its experimental genre in particular.

One of the two principal branches of ethics, in philosophy, is characterized as being *teleological* (Gr. *telos*, 'end') in its fundamental principle: a chosen action is ethical if it is intended to maximize the aggregate of happiness among those who are affected by it. In teleological terms, thus, for a planned epidemiological experiment on the effect of some intervention on the population level to be ethical, required is, first, that the study's design – as for both objects and methods – is, as best the investigators can tell (upon all the necessary inputs and reflections), free of recognized errors; second, that its execution will be made as flawless as possible; and third, that the resulting advancement in the knowledge-base of epidemiological practice is expected to enhance human happiness more than the study subjects' participation in the trial, together with whatever other 'costs' of the trial, will take away from it. The operative criterion of teleological ethics indeed is this *sincere effort* to choose the course of action that maximizes the aggregate happiness of those who will be affected by the study, *not success* in this effort. An epidemiological experiment on humans thus is not teleologically unethical just because it produced only unhappiness (due to, e.g., some common misunderstanding in the study's objects' design; sects. 7.2, 7.3).

The other principal branch of ethics, in philosophy, is characterized as being *deontological* (Gr. *deon*, 'binding'). It seeks to define ethical *obligations*, duties. As for human experimentation in epidemiological (and other) research, the overarching ethical obligation, now strictly binding to the researchers, has to do with the study subjects' *informed consent* to the participation: without such consent from each of the study subjects, the study is deontologically unethical. This is commonly accompanied by deontological guidelines for the maintenance of *confidentiality* of the information collected on the study subjects.

Informed consent in intervention-prognostic research on humans is commonly thought of as pertaining, specifically, to each study subject's *enrollment* into a trial, with experts' *equipoise* about the interventions' relative merits seen to be an added prerequisite for ethical solicitation of the enrollment; but both of these ideas are *untenable*, arguably at least.

As the decision to enter into a trial is to be an informed one, so logically should also be continued participation in it, notably when new information accrues from the study itself and/or from concomitant other studies: the information for the consent should be updated, as indicated. But as it now is, the trial's Data Safety and Monitoring Board or its equivalent, in the light of merely the accruing data in the trial itself and in the context of its own valuations, periodically decides to continue the trial until, perhaps, abruptly calling it to a halt (notably as, suddenly, there is a statistically significant difference, as $P < \alpha$).

And equipoise, insofar as it should be seen to be relevant at all, should be that of each potential study subject, whose subjective valuations matter in addition to whatever objective information is supplied by experts. But actually, a potential study subject should be free to volunteer for the advancement of the knowledge-base of the practice of epidemiology (sect. 1.1) even in the face of whatever disutility this action may subjectively seem to entail to the volunteer. By the same token, there should not be any deontological prohibition of solicitation of participation in an experiment, given provision of all of the relevant information about it. After all, the investigator's experimentation on him- or herself is not being considered to be ethically inadmissible (see sect. 12.3).

Overall, the ethics of human experimentation in epidemiological research remains incompletely developed even in respect to its broadest principles, and much could be said about disingenuous heeding of such ethical – deontological – norms as generally are being formally upheld.

9.5   Quasi-experimental Intervention Studies

The implementation of an intervention experiment in population-level epidemiological research is, commonly, quite challenging, from the recruitment of volunteers for enrollment into the study cohort through all the necessary work on it as for intervention execution and data collection – commonly over a long period of time, inescapably prospective from the vantage of the trial's initiation.

This raises the question of whether intervention effects really need to be studied in the framework of experimental simulation of practice, instead of setting out to learn from experiences in actual practice, documented for the purposes of practice (rather than science) – given that the compared interventions actually are being used in actual practice.

In contemplating this alternative to experimentation, it is to be borne in mind that the objects of epidemiological intervention studies have a particular structure (sect. 9.2); and that, consequently, the intervention studies themselves have a structure characteristic of them (sect. 9.3.).

The question about possible non-experimental alternatives to intervention experiments in population-level epidemiological research thus takes this form: Can *quasi-experimental* alternatives to those experiments, when distinctly more feasible to construct, also be without appreciable compromise of validity? Such studies would be, by definition, like their experimental counterparts as for the structure of them, but they would not actually be experiments in terms of that which is definitional to intervention experiments as distinct from their quasi-experimental counterparts: the genesis of this structure, specifically the adoptions of the interventions for the (sole) purpose of learning about their effects (sect. 9.1).

In quasi-experimental intervention studies the interventions are ones adopted so as to elicit their already known, or at least presumed, intended effects. In these, the intervention-study structure is achieved not by constructing it but, instead, by suitable *selection* of the study subjects so as to achieve the needed structure – as though an experimental protocol had been followed.

The central reservation about quasi-experimental intervention studies relates, naturally, to the very feature that makes them only *quasi*-experimental in the study of *intended* effects (of interventions). Non-experimental, non-randomized studies of the intended effects of alternative interventions are prone to be subject to incompletely documentable and, hence, less than adequately controllable *confounding by indication* in studies of the interventions' intended effects, notably when used are data recorded for the purposes of actual practice (rather than for research).

Ill-documented particulars of the indication's severity bear on the risk of the outcome at issue, and they may also have differential bearing on the choice of intervention. This problem of potentially uncontrollable confounding by indication generally is, however, much lesser in epidemiological research on preventive interventions than in clinical research on therapeutic interventions, on account of the generally simpler indications in the former.

Quasi-experimental intervention studies do have their place in the development of the scientific knowledge-base of epidemiological practice, and the place is characterized by *simple indication* for *acute interventions* and interest in *long-term effects* of these, so long as the alternative interventions have been in use for long-enough period of time.

Chapter 10
Causal Studies' Acausal Counterparts

Abstract In community-level preventive medicine the core mission of reducing morbidity from various illnesses involves two principal components: reduction of the occurrence of causes of illnesses and reduction of people's susceptibilities to such causes as remain.

When decisions about these actions – quitting smoking or undergoing vaccination, for example – are taken by individual members of the cared-for population – in response to community-level health education – people's rational decisions about them require *assessments of their personal risks* for the illnesses that are at issue. Insofar as the knowledge-base for this is available – from population-level epidemiological research, acausal/descriptive – individuals in the cared-for population can perform their personal risk assessments on the basis of a web-based system arranged by the health educators.

The knowledge-base of these risk assessments is constituted by *risk functions*. For a given one of these, the domain is one in which the risk assessment is done, and subdomains within this are defined by risk/prognostic indicators for the health outcome at issue. The risk function, thus, expresses the cumulative probability of the health event's occurrence over prospective/prognostic time as a function of that time (T) jointly with the prognostic indicators at the time of the risk assessment (at prognostic T_0). The risk function is predicated on no change in the risk factors (causal) over the time horizon addressed by the function.

In an acausal prognostic study, as in an intervention-prognostic study, a cohort is enrolled from the risk function's domain of application, and the study base is formed by this cohort's prospective course (away from the domain of application). A case series from this study base is coupled with an unstratified sample of this population-time, to be able to assess incidence-density function subject to translation into the corresponding function for cumulative incidence – and hence risk – from T_0 to T.

O.S. Miettinen and I. Karp, *Epidemiological Research: An Introduction*,
DOI 10.1007/978-94-007-4537-7_10, © Springer Science+Business Media Dordrecht 2012

10.1   The Focus on Prevention-oriented Research

Epidemiological practice has traditionally been *public-health medicine* in the principal meaning of *community-level preventive medicine*, the broadest modalities in this being education, regulation, and service. This community segment of preventive practice has been supplemented by clinical preventive medicine, while preventive medicine at large has been supplemented – backed up – by therapeutic and rehabilitative clinical medicine.

Accordingly, a secondary concern in community health-education has been optimization of people's deployment of clinical care – prevention of its underuse and, also, overuse. In his *Tracking Medicine: A Researcher's Quest to Understand Health Care* (2010), John Wennberg makes an evidence-based case for overuse of available healthcare being counterproductive to population health: "Our research finds support for [the hypothesis that] greater care intensity is associated with higher mortality rates and poorer objective measures of process quality" (p. 160).

In the modern context of *national health insurance*, clinical medicine, too, has become a component in public-health medicine, in fact the principal component by far; and this has substantially enlarged the scope of epidemiological practice of public-health medicine. In the main this new segment of epidemiological practice is a matter of something other than preventive medicine; it is documentation of rates of occurrence of phenomena of care providers' actions within the jurisdiction of the epidemiologist's concern, for clinicians' evaluation of the quality of the care and possible corrective actions by administrative and/or policy-making officials. This fact-finding, addressed in section 14.5, is commonly misconstrued as research and termed health services research.

As epidemiological practice thus interfaces with clinical practice, its knowledge-base has a partial overlap with that of clinical medicine. From this it does not follow, however, that epidemiological research (scientific) should extend beyond what is needed for the scientific knowledge-base of community-level preventive medicine. For, whatever the community doctor needs to know about clinical medicine – about screening for a cancer (ch. 11), for example – (s)he can and should obtain from the relevant clinicians.

Community medicine in the form of service can be a matter of preventive intervention on individuals dealt with one at a time, as in clinical medicine. Community projects/programs of vaccination are prime examples of this. But there are no corresponding community-level projects or programs of therapeutic or rehabilitative services, as these – like vaccinations – need to be provided individually but never indiscriminately – different from vaccinations.

The outlook in play here – in terms of which individuals in the cared-for population take personal decisions in the light of what they have come to understand are their individualized risks and the susceptibilities of these for reduction, and their personal valuations of these – is no different from that in clinical medicine, whether preventive or therapeutic. But we must point out that in a very eminent little book, *The Strategy of Preventive Medicine* (1992), Jeffrey Rose – this highly esteemed professor of epidemiology – argued otherwise. He accented the importance of the cumulative effect on the population level of even minor gains by the individuals involved. In this book's Preface he wrote, "The essential determinants of health of society are thus to be found in mass characteristics: ... effective prevention requires changes which involve the population as a whole."

10.2 The Acausal Knowledge-base of Prevention ·

Women in the population that an epidemiologist serves do not look for guidance from the epidemiologist's health-education in respect to reduction of their risks for prostate cancer; but they do look for guidance in respect to prevention of coronary heart disease and stroke, for example. Interest in, and relevance of, prevention-oriented measures of maintenance of low-risk lifestyle naturally depends on the perceived level of risk for the illness at issue. An epidemiologist's health-education thus needs to provide for *individual risk assessments* in the community (s)he serves.

While rate inherently is a population-level concept in epidemiology, *risk* inherently has to do with individuals (as members of a population perhaps). Risk is, for an individual, the probability – in the objective, relative frequency meaning of this – that the outcome – adverse – at issue will come about. It inherently is conditional on whatever is the known *risk profile* – prognostic profile – of the particular person at the time of the risk assessment, the prognostication in this sense. The (profile-conditional) probability/risk of the outcome's occurrence is defined in reference to a particular *risk period* for this, and it is the proportion of instances of the risk profile in general – in the abstract – such that the outcome will occur within this period. Risk per se is *acausal*, having to do with this proportion conditionally on a particular intervention (such as none) with no causal contrast involved. It also is, for scholarly purposes at least, conditional on surviving extraneous causes of death over the risk period at issue.

In preventive medicine, risk assessment is relevant for decisions about prevention-oriented actions in two stages. The first stage is assessment of *background risk*, meaning risk conditional on no (new) prevention-oriented action – no change in, say, dietary habits. And if this risk is assessed and deemed high enough to entertain such a change, *change-conditional* risks also need to be assessed – for assessment of the changes in risk over various periods that would result from the action being considered. These two types of risk, considered jointly in respect to a given potential action on the part of a particular individual at a particular time, imply the causal *risk difference* relevant to the decision about the action.

10.3   The Objects of the Acausal Studies

The generic object of study for risk assessments with a view to potential prevention-oriented action, for individuals' decisions about the action, is a *risk function* designed for a defined *domain* of risk assessment. This function may address the risk conditionally on no action (preventive), or the risk may be formulated as a function also of a potential action/ inaction with a view to the individualized risk difference by the action, reflecting the effect (preventive) of this action when adopted in lieu of no action.

Regardless of whether potential prevention-oriented action is involved, the risk is modeled as a function of *prognostic indicators* relevant to consider as definers of subdomains of the function's domain; and the function generally needs to define the risk not for a single risk period but as a function of *prognostic time* – as to the form of those functional dependencies of the risk.

10.4   The Acausal Studies Proper

An experiment ('trial') designed to address the effectiveness of a prevention-oriented intervention inherently provides for addressing intervention-conditional risk functions (sect. 9.3); and by the same token, the corresponding quasi-experiments (sect. 9.5) also do.

Ordinarily, a risk-assessment study involves enrollment a cohort of study subjects as representatives of the domain of risk assessment, from among candidates for the enrollment identified in a chosen source population. For efficiency of study, the enrollment is selective with a view to increasing the variability of the prognostic indicators' realizations at entry into the study cohort. At entries into the cohort, at cohort and prognostic T_0, the study subjects' prognostic profiles are documented. And following the entries, the cohort members are followed principally with a view to identifying and documenting the 'end point' of the follow-up, the illness event at issue. The empirical counterpart of the designed risk function is derived from the resulting data as discussed in section 9.3.

That is the essence of the study so long as studied is the risk in the absence of any knowledge about measures to prevent the illness, ones that might be applied by the study subjects in the course of the follow-up. And it also is the study's essence when an added feature is (random) assignments to particular ones of prevention-oriented interventions, together with implementations/enforcements and documentations of these (sect. 9.3). Otherwise the study is tantamount to a quasi-experimental intervention study, with its challenges in validity assurance (sect. 9.5).

An intervention-conditional, acausal risk function should be not only valid/unbiased but also maximally discriminating among different levels of risk within the study objects' domain. As a measure of the empirical function's discriminatingness/*informativeness*, some use the area under the ROC (receiver operator characteristic) curve.

More meaningful as a measure of a risk function's informativeness (validity-conditional) might be taken to the standard deviation of the function-based risk values divided by the maximum that this SD could possibly be. Empirically, this informativeness index is

$$\hat{I} = \left[\hat{V} \Big/ \frac{N}{N-1} \hat{R} \left(1 - \hat{R} \right) \right]^{1/2},$$

where, based on a representative cohort from the function's domain, $\hat{V}$ is the unbiased 'estimate' of the unit variance of the N values of risk from the function and $\hat{R}$ is the empirical value for the unconditional risk (proportion with $Y = 1$) among the N instances.

Chapter 11
Studies on Screening for a Cancer

Abstract An epidemiologist's concern for the health of the cared-for community/population actually is not limited to community-level preventive medicine, without regard for whatever may be going on in the clinical segment of healthcare at large. (S)he understands that the people's health – public health in this meaning of the term – is much influenced by the aggregate of clinical healthcare (preventive, therapeutic, rehabilitative) in the community – mostly for the better but, also, for the worse. And as a consequence, (s)he is concerned to optimize people's use of clinical care by means of *community-level health education aimed at prevention of both under- and overuse of clinical care*.

One line of this education has to do with *screening for risk factors* for illnesses (e.g., the BRCA 1 & 2 mutations with a view to detection of high risk for breast cancer), preparatory to decision about preventive interventions (e.g., by tamoxifen use) and/or *screening for the illness* at issue (breast cancer in this example) – that is, pursuit of early, latent-stage diagnosis (rule-in) about the illness with a view to enhanced curability by early treatment.

Screening is directed to individuals one at a time, and it thus is *clinical* healthcare, by definition. Screening for a risk factor is *preventive* care, while screening for an illness is *therapeutic* – therapy-oriented – care (when opportunity for successful prevention already is passé). The yield of screening is *information*, and this in itself has no effect on the person's course of health. It thus is not an intervention.

This chapter addresses, in the main, the epidemiologic researchers' *misunderstandings* in regard to these orientational concepts and the consequent serious misunderstandings about research on the intended consequences of screening, for a cancer in particular. Epidemiologists should come to understand that the knowledge-base, just as practice, of screening is a *clinical* matter.

O.S. Miettinen and I. Karp, *Epidemiological Research: An Introduction*,   113
DOI 10.1007/978-94-007-4537-7_11, © Springer Science+Business Media Dordrecht 2012

11.1   Introductory Example

The risk for breast cancer – overt, life-threatening cancer of a breast – is very high for women with certain exceptional – mutant BRCA 1 and/or BRCA 2 – genes. This topic is of considerable healthcare concern, as screening for these very major risk factors is practicable, as effective preventive interventions (by tamoxifen use or even by bilateral mastectomy) are available options, and as screening for the cancer (with a view to enhanced curability) is practicable – all of this, naturally, in *clinical* medicine.

Even though this care is, by its very nature, a matter of clinical, rather than community, medicine, it nevertheless is a concern from the vantage of *public health* and its attendant public policies, now that clinical healthcare has been brought to the public domain via the advent of national health insurance. On the other hand, though, the promulgators of the public policies are constrained by the 'social contract' that leaves the medical professions autonomous – free of societal domination – in specifically medical aspects of the care.

This topic differs quite profoundly from the ones addressed in section 4.1 in that the public policies about it are not legalistic-regulatory and directed to the public's behaviors or environments outside the realm of (professional) healthcare. They are, instead, directed to the relevant healthcare (clinical), by physicians. But consistent with autonomy of the medical professions, the public policies are not normative stipulations concerning the care; they are about societal *reimbursements* of the costs of the care.

So, what do the promulgators of healthcare policies (on reimbursements) principally need to know about clinical care related to this genetic aspect of breast cancer? and how will they get to know it? It is relevant to note first, in the particular context here for a start, that they do not need to know about the etiogenetic proportions for those genotypes in cases of breast cancer associated with those genotypes, from causal research of the etiogenetic genus. The frequency – prevalence – of each of those genotypes is a matter not of human behavior (unpredictable, capricious, as in the first three of the four examples in sect. 4.1) nor of people's environments (also quite variable) but of human biology, and these rates are knowable from genetical-epidemiological research. But again, policy promulgators need not know about these proportions either.

Instead, the policy-makers' need is to know about the risk of coming down with overt breast cancer – say, life-time cumulative risk of this – among women with those genetic traits, this naturally from descriptive, acausal research for risk assessment (ch. 10). And in particular, the policy-makers need to know much more from specifically *clinical research* so as to have the scientific basis, supplemented by economic facts, for assessing the *cost-effectiveness* of the care, this being central to the perceived justifiability/unjustifiability of societal reimbursement of its cost.

11.2   Epidemiologists' Outlook

Concerning a particular generic type of *cancer* – breast or lung cancer, say – epidemiologists' concern generally does not focus on the rate of incidence of diagnosis (first rule-in dgn.) about it, nor on the rate of the cancer's prevalence, but, instead, on the rate of incidence of death from it – on *mortality* from the cancer, that is.

The concern being reduction of that mortality (by community-oriented means), one avenue to this end is promotion of *early detection* of the cancer, this on the premise that provision for early treatment provides for more common cures of the cancer and, thereby, reduction in mortality from it. This is a matter of promoting *screening* for the cancer – pursuit of diagnosis (rule-in dgn.) about the cancer in its preclinical, latent stage of development, *baseline* screening followed by periodic *repeat* screenings. This promotion is adopted into epidemiological practice in regard to a particular segment of the cared-for population as a matter of *public policy* if the screening in this subpopulation is deemed to produce enough life-saving – mortality-reducing – benefit to justify its attendant harm and monetary cost.

In this promotion there are two fundamental options. One option is community education focusing on the screening in the framework of clinical medicine, while an alternative to this is internal to community medicine: community education about, and community-level provision of, the initial testing, with referral of the test-positive persons for further diagnostic work-up in the clinical framework (together with early treatment in the event of the cancer's rule-in dgn.).

Epidemiologists' preference, at present, generally is for the latter; and associated with this is *viewing community-level provision of the first diagnostic test as a community-level intervention*, and a *preventive* (*sic*) intervention at that (Apps. 1, 2). From this major fallacy is deduced the idea that study of the mortality-reducing effectiveness of screening is, ideally at least, a matter of *randomized trials* – and, notably, clinical (*sic*) trials at that.

Three features generally characterize epidemiologists' *design of these trials*, quite regularly touted as representing the 'gold standard' in this research: arbitrary (and commonly very small) number of repeat screenings; attention to deaths from the cancer throughout an arbitrary duration of follow-up (post randomization); and disregard for the timings of these deaths by focus on single-valued proportional reduction (apparent) in mortality from the cancer over the duration (arbitrary) of the follow-up (cf. sect. 7.2). As the community-level 'intervention' on any given individual never extends beyond the initial test, yet another feature of these trials generally is absence of any protocol for the rest of the diagnostic work-up and for the treatment upon diagnosis (rule-in) about the cancer.

11.3 The 'Gold Standard' Trial

A hypothetical example of a screening 'intervention' experiment, for simplicity focusing on the mortality implications of the *baseline* round of screening for a cancer, is addressed in Table 11.1 here. More specifically, of course, the focus in this special case of the 'gold standard' study on screening for a cancer is on mortality from cases of the cancer – latent cases – that are *detectable* by the screening (by the baseline version of its regimen/protocol or by the aggregate of the corresponding unregimented practices; cf. above). At issue is early detection (under screening) versus no early detection (under no screening), mortality in relation to this.

According to that table, its Part A, the fatalities from those detectable cases in the absence of screening-based early detection occur 2-12 years later; 10% 2-4 years later, 30% 4-6 years later, and 60% 6-12 years later. And that Part A of the table also shows that of the potential fatalities in those three successive periods of prospective time, 10, 40, and 90%, respectively, are preventable by screening-associated early treatments. (The later is the potential death from the cancer, the earlier is the cancer's stage of development at the time of the potential screening; and as a consequence, the later is the potential fatality, the greater is the cancer's curability – and the death's consequent preventability – by early treatment.)

Part B of that table shows the implications of the time-specific preventability rates – by early treatment – in otherwise fatal (but detectable) cases, implied by Part A. The focus is on the reduction in *cumulative* mortality, separately for the cases that are detectable by screening at baseline and for these cases in combination with those that are not yet detectable at the time of the baseline screening. While the former proportional reductions are shown to be, at 6, 12, and 20 years, 13, 69, and 69, respectively, the latter ones are less than 13%, much less than 69%, and very much less than 69%, respectively.

Table 11.1 Hypothetical example concerning *baseline* screening

Part A. Fatality implications of the screening (of its associated early trmt) in cases detectable at baseline

Detectable cases fatal under *no screening*: time to death	*Reduction* in detectable cases' fatal outcomes under screening[a]
<2 yr: 0%	<2 yr: –
2-4 yr: 10%	2-4 yr: 10%
4-6 yr: 30%	4-6 yr: 40%
>6 yr: 60%	>6 yr: 90%

Part B. Reduction in *cumulative* mortality

1. Baseline-detectable cases	2. Baseline- and *later*-detectable cases
6 yr: $0.1 \times 0.1 + 0.3 \times 0.4 = 13\%$	6 yr: <13%
12 yr: $0.13 + 0.6 \times 0.9 = 69\%$	12 yr: ≪69%
20 yr: 69%	20 yr: ≪≪69%

[a]This is the rate of *curability*, by early treatment, of otherwise fatal detectable cases

Now, insofar as one in this example wishes to think about screening-associated reduction in cumulative mortality from the cancer (consequent to early treatments), one must be thinking about the screen-detectable subset of the cases (as among the rest of the cases there is, at baseline, no screening-based reduction in the prospective fatal outcomes). In the example addressed in Table 11.1 here, this means that one's interest is focused on that 69% – the proportional reduction in otherwise fatal outcomes of the detectable cases.

That 69% reduction in fatalities from those baseline-detectable cases translates into the same reduction in the cumulative mortality from the cancer for that subset of cases at 12 years of follow-up and later (but not earlier) – but this reduction is *not manifest at any time* in the follow-up of screened and unscreened subcohorts in a randomized trial on the screening (baseline scr. vs. no scr.). Manifest in the trial's screening arm are only cumulative rates of mortality from the cancer for the baseline-detectable cases in combination with ones that only later become detectable (by repeat screening); the manifest reductions in the cumulative rate of mortality from the cancer are smaller than the curability rate of otherwise fatal cases, that 69%, at whatever time after the baseline screenings, some of them much smaller. (See Part B of Table 11.1.)

Upshot: *Nothing quantitatively meaningful is addressed in this 'gold-standard' trial on screening for a cancer* (the way they are designed; sect. 11.2 above).

11.4   Meaningful Types of Trial

As we repeatedly let on in the two sections above, screening for a cancer, in itself, does not reduce mortality from the cancer as, contrary to common claim, it is not an intervention. Only the screening-afforded early treatments (in lieu of later ones) have the potential for that consequence (in causal terms), on the ground of enhanced curability of otherwise fatal cases of the cancer.

And we also showed, in section 11.3 above, that this curability gain is not manifest in the proportional reduction in cumulative mortality from the cancer in such screening trials as ordinarily are designed and carried out; that such a mortality reduction generally grossly underrepresents the proportion of cases that are curable by early treatment among otherwise incurable, fatal cases of the cancer; that, in fact, nothing quantitatively meaningful is studyable by means of such trials. And qualitatively, the mere existence of the reduction generally should be understood not to be a hypothesis but a corollary of the attainability of earlier, latent-stage diagnosis and the enhanced curability consequent to this.

Harkening back, again, to the example in section 10.3 above, that curability rate (69%) for early-detected, otherwise fatal cases obviously is, in principle, studyable by means of an actual *intervention trial*. In it, some of the baseline screen-detected cases (a random subset) of the cancer would be treated without delay, others only if and when they progress to overt, symptomatic disease.

In the absence of any 'overdiagnoses' – taking practically benign lesions to be life-threatening – the relative magnitudes of the cumulative incidence of death from the cancer in the trial's two arms, once leveling off (after 12 years of follow-up), would obviously give an empirical measure of the proportion of the cases such that only early treatment is life-saving. And as a matter of fact, even if there would be overdiagnosis, these asymptotic levels of the cumulative incidence would not need to be corrected for the proportion of overdiagnosed cases (the frequency of which could be studied on the basis of the delayed-treatment arm of the trial) in order that their relative magnitudes fairly represent the curability gain from the screening-associated early diagnoses.

That type of trial would be quite straightforward, as the focus would be on the true causal contrast – not screening versus no screening but early, latent-stage treatment versus treatment delayed until the disease is overt, symptomatic – and addressed would be the contrasted treatments' relative effects – preventive – on all of the cancer's naturally fatal outcomes, across all of their timings, and without admixture of deaths from cases of the cancer outside the causal contrast (cf. sect. 11.3).

In these terms, study of reduction in mortality from the cancer – in the meaning of case-fatality rate – would be meaningful, completely so, separately for baseline and repeat screenings. But of course, recruitment of well-informed volunteers would tend to present a practically insurmountable problem of feasibility.

A randomized *screening trial* is profoundly different from that screening-related intervention trial. It contrasts screening with no screening; and while it generally has been quantitatively meaningless (if not downright misleading and grossly so; sect. 11.3), with proper design and its corresponding execution it too would be properly informative about the curability gain and its consequent mortality reduction attendant to the cancer's early detection. But the requirements are quite onerous, and it is important to appreciate that even an ideal trial of this type – just like the intervention trial above – can never meaningfully address the mortality consequence of the screening's introduction into a community. Both of these topics we address below.

For an RST to be quantitatively meaningful, there needs to be a segment in the cohort time of follow-up such that all members of the screened subcohort have, in this period, histories of full survival benefit of the screenings (periodic) – really, to say it again, of screening-associated early treatment of the cancer. It is in that segment of the trial's cohort time that the screened subcohort's mortality from the cancer is reduced to the extent – in the proportion – that the early interventions cure otherwise fatal cases of the cancer.

Harkening, again, back to the example (hypothetical) in section 11.3 above, the mortality-reducing consequence of the *baseline* screening (with no screening as the alternative) occurs, completely, in the cohort time interval of 2–12 years (after the cohort T_0, the time of the randomization to the baseline screening, only , or to no screening); only in this period of time could the baseline screening bear on the cancer's outcome. But in this segment of the cohort time the attained rate of cures at baseline, in otherwise fatal cases, is not manifest in (the complement of) the ratio of the cumulative rates of mortality from the cancer (in one minus this ratio), as included in the screened-arm experience are deaths from cases that only subsequently were detectable – but were not detected – by the screening. The mortality ratio in this segment of follow-up is, thus, substantially 'diluted' toward unity (from the $1.00 - 0.69 = 0.31$; cf. sect. 11.3 above).

Now, consider an RST that involves also regular *repeat* screenings – annual ones, say – and suppose the latent cases detectable by these screenings also would have their fatal outcomes 2-12 years following the detections in the absence of early treatment. In this RST there can be a period of follow-up time in which deaths from the cancer in the trial's screening arm are reduced by a proportion identical to the screening-associated rate of cures of otherwise fatal cases. This period, if there, *begins* at 12 years of follow-up on the condition that *the screening's duration* exceeds $12 - 2 = 10$ years; and the length of this period is the same as the duration of that exceedance.

In this period of maximal reduction in the mortality, if it exists (by the duration of the screening), all deaths from the cancer in the trial's screening arm are associated with a history of diagnosis under the screenings – repeat screenings – and their associated early treatment. The diagnoses about these cases were either screening-based or prompted by symptoms appearing between scheduled screenings. In these cases the early diagnosis – its associated treatment – failed to halt the cancer's progression to its fatal outcome.

Addressed in the foregoing has been study of the extent of a cancer's enhanced curability by means of experimental experience with the way case-fatality rate from the cancer is affected by screening (by its associated early treatments). With this *clinical* matter settled (more or less), the genuinely *epidemiological* question remains, as it is about the mortality consequence of the introduction of a public-health program to reduce the deaths' incidence density (sect. 11.2). The program could be one of mere reimbursement of the cost of the initial test in the diagnostics constituting the screening, coupled with education of the public about the screening (in the clinical domain); or it could be education about, and provision of, community-level service as a matter of providing the screening's initial testing (sect. 11.2).

So, the research – clinical research – outlined above actually is about curability implications of mortality experience with experimental screening, while the question relevant to epidemiological practice is about the *mortality implications of that curability*, this in reference to the contemplated public-health program(s). This question is *not addressed* by this research – nor is it subject to being answered by any epidemiological research. But to the extent – depending on indications and quality assurance – the screening is clinically justified, it also is public-health-justified, now that clinical medicine, too, is public-health medicine (given national health insurance). For more on these challenging matters, see Appendix 2.

11.5 Meaningful Etiologic-type Study

Lack of screening for a cancer (of its associated early treatment) is etio-
logic/etiogenetic to death from the cancer. The extent to which this is so naturally
is studyable only where the screening has been available (but not routinely used).
And it is studyable to learn about the here-essential parameter of Nature – the
curability gain from screening-based early diagnoses – only in settings in which the
screening has been *available long enough*.

These opportune settings – ones in which the screening-afforded gain in curability could be quantified by means of etiogenetic studies – already are quite common;
and they really should be made use of for this purpose, for the serious problems
inherent in the 'gold standard' trials in this quantification (sects. 7.2, 11.3, 11.4) are
not shared by their etiogenetic counterparts.

The *study base* needs to be defined (as to age, i.a.) in such a way that associated
with each person-moment in it there was an opportunity for the screening in the
relevant past, 2–12 years ago in the example in section 11.3 above. Thus, if the
cancer at issue in this example is that of breast and it was introduced over 12 years
ago to women 50–70 years of age and has continued to be available only to women
in this range of age, the study base needs to be restricted to women 62–72 years of
age; for, women younger than 62 years of age did not have access to screening as
long as 12 years ago, and women more than 72 years of age did not have that access
as recently as two years ago. If the screening for that range of age was introduced
less than 12 years ago, no-one in the population had access to the screening for the
entire period of 2–12 years ago, so that a valid study base cannot yet be defined in
this setting.

For the *case series* (of death from the cancer, in a suitably defined study base
as to age, i.a.), the *index history* need not be that of regular screening throughout
the period of 2–12 years prior to the death (to continue the example). A sufficient
substitute for this has to do with the time of the cancer's diagnosis (rule-in dgn.): at
the time of the diagnosis the person was under screening, so that the diagnosis either
resulted from screening or was a symptoms-prompted interim diagnosis within a
regular-type cycle of the screening. (Additional screenings outside this particular
cycle could not have had any potential role in prevention of the death, so that
history about those screenings is irrelevant in the definition of the index history.)
The corresponding *reference history* in the case series is: diagnosis while not under
screening; that is, diagnosis not preceded by on-schedule initial test, with negative
result of the screening.

Definition of the index history for the *base series* presents the challenge that there
is no counterpart for the routine positive history of diagnosis (rule-in) about the
cancer in the case series, no inherently corresponding time on which to focus it and,
consequently, the reference history also. The solution of choice to this dilemma is
to use the case series as the guide to this timing: as a case (of death from the cancer)
has occurred at a particular time in age and calendar time, this prompts a number of
probes into the study base, into the same stratum of time (age and calendar time);

and for this set of person-moments in the study base, the screening history is defined in reference to the same time at which the first manifestation of the cancer (positive test result, or symptom) occurred in the member of the case series.

With the case series from the source base restricted to the limited range of age that is to characterize the study base (see above) and with the base series time-matched to this, another restriction also is of note here. Study of the curability gain requires that only one detected case of the cancer characterizes the histories in the case series, with none the counterpart of this in the base series.

If this is all that is in the scientific essence of the study design, then the data from the study lead to a set of 2×2 tables, each specific to a confounder stratum at the time of the outcome:

I	R	Total
c_{1j}	c_{0j}	C_j
b_{1j}	b_{0j}	B_j

where I and R denote the index and reference history (of screening), respectively, and C_j and B_j are the stratum-specific sizes of the case and base series, respectively (cf. sect. 5.4). And the confounder-adjusted empirical measure of the rate ratio (for death from the cancer, contrasting I with R) is

$$\widehat{RR}^* = \sum_j c_{1j} / \sum_j \left(b_{1j} c_{0j} / b_{0j} \right)$$

(cf. sect. 5.4); and the corresponding empirical measure of the *curability gain* from a round of screening (from screen diagnoses when added to interim diagnoses within the round) is the complement of this, $1 - \widehat{RR}^*$.

If the data are examined separately by categories of the etiogenetic time (retrospective as of the outcomes in the two series), presumably the $\widehat{RR}$s for more distant times are seen to be lower than those for more recent times (see Table 11.1 in sect. 11.3). This, while true, is irrelevant for the quantification of the curability gain so long as the rate of the screening's use has been essentially constant over that range of retrospective time – as evinced by the I/R ratio in the reference series over that span of time. Otherwise averaging of the time-specific RRs – their logarithms – is called for, with the $\widehat{RR}^*$ the antilog of this average (unweighted).

The foregoing implicitly involves the premise of no *confounding* in the study base according to extraneous determinants other than calendar time and age of the incidence density of death from the cancer. But insofar as there is, in the study base, potential confounding by other factors, they need to be accounted for in the model for the incidence density and, accordingly, in the logistic model fitted to the data – perhaps leading to stratification according to a confounder score (sect. 5.4).

As this is a non-experimental study on causation (of the etiogenetic sort), the question is, as always in this genre of studies, whether *all* of the potential confounders were identified and adequately documented, for control in the synthesis of the data to the result of the study. Now, undergoing a round of screening or refraining from this is a purposive course of action, and the indications of risk bearing on the decision about this action are known to the decision-makers and hence knowable to the investigators. The question is, though, whether the facts about these can validly be ascertained for both of the study series – from the next of kin in both of them.

In closing here, the comparative big picture. If a *randomized screening trial* is designed for long-enough continuation of the screening and the mortality contrast is focused on the right segment of follow-up time, it is still prone to produce a highly downward-biased empirical value for the curability gain – due to poor adherence to the assigned long-term screening and non-screening. In an *etiogenetic study*, such as was outlined above, the principal challenge in validity assurance is confounding by indication (for the screening), due to absence of randomization. But such residual confounding as on this basis will characterize the result is *negative confounding*, again biasing the empirical value of the curability gain downward – but much less so than the bias from the best possible screening trial.

   This leads to the need to appreciate fusion of these two types of study: when the experimental practice in an RST has continued long enough, this trial's population-time of follow-up constitutes a suitable source base for an etiogenetic study such as was outlined here – yielding a result less biased than the one from the right segment of the follow-up in the 'intention-to-screen' spirit of the trial, as the bias from the (quite considerable) non-adherence to the protocol is avoided.

   But as it is at present, reviews tend to focus on the RSTs alone; and in this, they tend to produce derivative results on mortality reduction as though the same parameter value were assessed with whatever duration of the screening and follow-up, and with no regard for the non-adherence to the contrasted regimens of screening versus non screening. See Appendix 2.

Chapter 12
Some Paradigmatic Studies

Abstract Thomas Kuhn, the eminent historiographer of science, is particularly well known for his description of the role of "paradigms" and "paradigm shifts" in science, especially in sciences in which eminent controversies are common – social science and psychology, in particular. Paradigms, he says, are "model problems" and "model solutions" that centrally influence research in the framework of "normal science." Along this path there is prone to develop a "crisis," leading to "revolutional science" and its associated new paradigm(s).

In chapter 2 it became evident that modern 'chronic-disease' epidemiological research is, in respect to such central "problems" as nutritional etiogenesis of cardiovascular disease and cancer, and the intended consequences of screening for a cancer, highly controversial about the implications of the accrued, very extensive evidence. Arguably at least, however, epidemiological research is, now, in a Kuhnian crisis – even though this is not commonly being recognized by the community of researchers concerned with problems of community medicine. As for model "problems," screening for a cancer continues to be viewed as a topic – quite eminent – in purportedly epidemiological (rather than clinical) research. And the controversies of social science may come to add to those endogenous to the biomedical research on the etiogenesis of illness, now that 'social epidemiology' is on the ascendency.

Population-level epidemiological research does lend itself to normal-science paradigms in respect to theory, but the prevailing methodologic ones are in need of revisions while paradigms of the studies' objects design are not only underdeveloped but in all essence non-existent. The randomized trial adopted from clinical research into epidemiological intervention studies is, now, a very false paradigm for research on screening for a cancer, having earlier been a false paradigm of the 'cohort' study on etiogenesis.

O.S. Miettinen and I. Karp, *Epidemiological Research: An Introduction*,
DOI 10.1007/978-94-007-4537-7_12, © Springer Science+Business Media Dordrecht 2012

While paradigms for research are important and tenable paradigms are particularly desirable, they should not be seen to define the boundaries of productive research. Some problems require extraparadigmatic solutions, even ones worthy of Nobel Prize for Physiology and Medicine.

12.1   The Role of Paradigmatic Studies

A student preparing for a career in epidemiological research will do well studying some of the history and philosophy of science in general, orientationally through Thomas Kuhn's *The Structure of Scientific Revolutions* (1970).

Based on his review of the history of social and psychological as well as natural science, Kuhn adduces the concept of "normal science," defining it as "research firmly based upon one or more past scientific achievements, achievements that some particular scientific community acknowledges for a time as supplying the foundation for its further [studies]" (p. 10). He explains that: "Today such achievements are recounted, though seldom in their original form, by science textbooks, elementary and advanced. ... [These writings serve] for a time implicitly to define the legitimate problems and methods of a research field for succeeding generations of [researchers in the field]" (p. 10).

Such achievements, ones that "provide models from which spring particular coherent traditions of scientific research" Kuhn terms *paradigms* (p. 10). "Men whose research is based on shared paradigms are committed to the same rules and standards for scientific [research]. That commitment and the apparent consensus it produces are prerequisites for normal science, i.e., for the genesis and continuation of a particular tradition" (p. 11).

"History suggests that the road to a firm research consensus is extraordinarily arduous" (p. 11). Thus, "fundamental disagreements characterized, for example, the study of motion before Aristotle and of statics before Archimedes, the study of heat before Black, of chemistry before Boyle and Boerhaave, and of historical geology before Hutton. In parts of biology – the study of heredity, for example – the first universally received paradigms are still more recent; and it remains an open question what parts of social science have yet achieved such paradigms at all" (p. 11).

Once a paradigm – "an accepted model or pattern" (p. 23) – has come into being, "it is an object for further articulation and specification under new or more stringent conditions" (p. 23).

Researchers in a given field of science "agree in their *identification* of a paradigm without agreeing on, or even attempting, to produce, a full *interpretation* or *rationalization* of it. Lack of a standard interpretation or of an agreed reduction to rules will not prevent a paradigm from guiding research" (p. 44; italics in the original). "Scientists work from models acquired through education and through subsequent exposure to the literature often without quite knowing or needing to know what characteristics have given these models the status of community paradigms" (p. 46).

"In the development of any science, the first received paradigm is usually felt to account quite successfully for most of the observations and experiments easily accessible to that science's [researchers]. Further development, therefore, ordinarily calls for the construction of elaborate equipment, the development of an esoteric vocabulary and skills, and a refinement of concepts that increasingly lessens their resemblance to their usual common-sense prototypes. That professionalization leads ... to an *immense restriction of the scientist's vision and to a considerable resistance to paradigm change*" (p. 64; italics ours).

12.2 Paradigmatic Causal Studies

In epidemiological research at present, normal-science paradigms dominate etiologic/etiogenetic research in terms of 'cohort' study and 'case-control' study in particular (sects. 2.6, 6.1, 6.2); intervention research in terms of randomized controlled trial (ch. 9); and screening research on a cancer also in terms of RCT (sect. 11.3).

The 'cohort' study and 'case-control' study are different not because of a corresponding difference in what is being studied; the distinction is merely methodologic. Yet the respective results appear to be different. Routinely reported from a 'cohort' study now is a result in terms of 'relative risk' or, alternatively, 'risk ratio' or 'rate ratio,' while reported from a 'case-control' study most commonly now is something quite peculiar to this type of study: 'odds ratio.'

From an RCT on an actual intervention the reported result now quite routinely is a 'hazard ratio,' while from an RCT on screening for a cancer the reported result is (proportional) 'reduction in mortality' (from the cancer, due to the screening; sects. 7.3, 11.3).

This illustrates what we quoted above as a general observation of Thomas Kuhn, when applied specifically to epidemiological researchers; they "agree in their *identification* of a paradigm without agreeing on, or even attempting to produce, a full *interpretation* or *rationalization* of it." As we have let on, we do not regard those paradigms, now generally treated as 'received truths,' as having a tenable rationale – for reasons that we have put forward (sects. 6.1, 6.2, 6.3, 6.4, 6.5, 9.3, 11.3) and leave for the reader "to weigh and consider" (Bacon; sect. 1.4).

Below, we sketch alternatives to those prevailing paradigms, all of them concerned with causal research. These sketches do not bring forth anything essential we haven't yet said or implied. Rather, they represent an attempt at crystallization of what we've already said, at concentration of the reader's mind on some essentials in introductory but nevertheless critical study of the theory of epidemiological research (cf. Preface).

We are, as has become apparent, of the mind that in *etiogenetic research* it is time for a 'paradigm shift' (Kuhn) away from the 'cohort' and 'case-control' studies, which we see as representing the cohort and trohoc fallacies, respectively (sects. 6.1, 6.2). We suggest replacement of these by a singular conception of the nature of (population-level) etiogenetic studies: *the* etiogenetic study (sect. 6.5).

As for *intervention research*, we can be seen to adhere to the prevailing, randomized-trial paradigm, except for a proposed modification of it. We propose that the object of the trial should not be a 'hazard ratio' but an intervention-prognostic probability function, and we delineate the way in which this can be studied in the framework of such data as already are routinely collected in these trials (sects. 9.2, 9.3).

Mass application of a screening test is taken to be an important type of intervention – preventive intervention – by epidemiologists and by promulgators of policies for healthcare (sect. 2.6, i.a.). For this reason we address *screening research* – specifically, research on screening for a cancer – in this book (ch. 11, i.a.). But we hold those ideas of epidemiologists and promulgators of healthcare policy to be mistaken, and screening for a cancer to be a topic – first and foremost a *diagnostic* topic – in *clinical* medicine (sects. 11.1, 11.2, i.a.). It is only because of that common misunderstanding that we address screening (for a cancer) in this book on epidemiological, rather than clinical, research. Further attention to it we give in Appendix 2.

Nutritional epidemiology was the principal focus in most of the chapter on epidemiological knowledge at present (ch. 2), due to the centrality of thinking about nutrition (incl. nutritional supplements) in modern preventive medicine – in industrialized countries in particular.

The big picture that emerged had these features of particular note here: nutritional etiology/etiogenesis of a phenomenon of health can be very chronic (as in, e.g., overt cases of various cancers) or quite acute (as in, e. g., weight gain); and research on nutritional etiogenesis of illness has had notable deficiencies in its objects designs in respect to the temporal aspect of the etiogenesis – and, also, in the formulation of the causal contrasts in the objects of study (chs. 2, 7).

A *paradigmatic*, exceptionally successful nutritional-etiogenetic study would be an experimental one. For, the causal contrasts in this research are too intricate (sect. 7.1) for proper documentation from non-experimental diets. Of course, only relatively short-term experimentation would be practicable, and the here-envisioned paradigmatic experiment thus is instructive about what hypotheses are, and which ones are not, subject to truly meaningful human-level testing. (Science does have its limits, and human experiments on, e.g., antioxidant deficiency in the etiogenesis of various cancers have been unrealistic and, hence, misleading; sects. 2.2, 7.1).

As Gary Taubes explains in his *Good Calories, Bad Calories* (2007), a practicable experiment, suitably designed and executed, could settle the now-so-topical, burning question about the dietary etiogenesis of weight gain and, hence, *obesity* – "whether it's excess calories that make us fat (the conventional wisdom) or purely the effect of carbohydrates on insulin and insulin on fat accumulation (the carbohydrate hypothesis)" (p. 466).

At issue is a *crucial experiment* with implications much beyond obesity: if the carbohydrate hypothesis is correct in respect to obesity, it thereby presumably is correct in respect to the genesis of the *'metabolic syndrome,'* seen to be at the root of obesity (sect. 2.4) and, independently of this, of many other illnesses besides: atheromatosis manifesting in cardiovascular disease (sect. 2.1); cancers (sect. 2.2); ageing (acceleration of its progression; sect. 2.3); dementias of old age (incl. Alzheimer's); 'hypertension' (sect. 2.5); and yet other illnesses too – as Taubes explains in that remarkable book (with the subtitle, "Fats, Carbs, and the Controversial Science of Diet and Health").

The paradigmatic study suggested here – the crucial experiment – would be about changes in *weight* and in level of *insulin* (and perhaps changes also in levels of glucose, triglycerides, and fractions of cholesterol) in 'blood' (plasma) over a span of time (months), in (sub)cohorts on different diets (randomly assigned) for that span of time. The study subjects' admissibility criteria would not be of critical importance to this study, but the definition of the set of diets would be.

The diets in this experiment would represent a contrast, for one, in the daily quantity of dietary energy intake conditional on the type-composition of the sources of energy (incl. beverages); and, conversely, there would be a type-composition contrast conditional on the quantity of energy. The paradigmatic experiment would, thus, represent a *factorial design* in this sense. The two levels of energy intake would represent an increased and the prevailing rate of energy intake, respectively; and the two type-compositions would represent an increased and the prevailing proportion of energy from carbohydrates.

The carbohydrate hypothesis about the etiogenesis of obesity that would be addressed by this study was widely, if not universally, held to be true until the 1970s (Taubes, p. 461), when the officially engineered shift away from fats in diets and correspondingly increased consumption of carbohydrates started in the U.S., followed by the major epidemic of obesity. The paradigmatic study just outlined – and in essence envisioned by Taubes (p. 466) – could re-establish the carbohydrate conception of the etiogenesis of obesity and many other 'diseases of civilization.'

12.3   Successful Extraparadigmatic Studies

A student being introduced into epidemiological research should not be left with the idea that hypotheses about etiology/etiogenesis derive solely from epidemiological studies on humans (with populations as units of observation perhaps; cf. sects. 2.1, 2.2, 2.6), or that testing of such hypotheses is best done by means of non-experimental etiogenetic study (sect. 6.5). The route to success may well be extraparadigmatic. In what follows, we illustrate this by the genesis of the idea that the etiogenesis of peptic ulcer involves a role for a bacterium.

The research, in Australia, that led to the discovery of the role of *Helicobacterium pylori* as the principal agent in the etiogenesis of peptic ulcer, gastric and duodenal, led the investigators to Stockholm, to receive the Nobel Prize. In outlining this research, we draw from – and direct the student to – two articles:

1. Van der Weyden M et alii. The 2005 Nobel Prize in physiology or medicine. *Med J Aust* 2005; 183: 612-4.
2. Atwood KC. Bacteria, ulcers, and ostracism? H. Pylori and the making of a myth. *Skeptical Inquirer Magazine* 2004; vol. 28.6. Available at: http://www. csicop.org/si/show/bacteria_ulcers_and_ostracism_h._pylori_and_the_making_of_ a_myth/. Accessed November 9, 2011.

The essentials of this research, according to reference 1 above, "illustrate some of the human hallmarks of revolutionary research. These include:

– being at the right place at the right time, and seeing what other people had seen but thinking of what nobody else thought [ref.];
– the role of serendipity;
– a passion for research that abandons personal safety with self-experimentation; and
– the inevitable resistance of the medical establishment as research undermines current dogma."

That last point is, however, disputed, seen to be a misrepresentation of what merely was the skepticism that is inherent in the scientific outlook (ref. 2).

Notable about the genesis of the hypothesis is that there were no insights from 'basic' science suggesting it, nor did the hypothesis arise from data on the occurrence of peptic ulcer in any human population. It arose from Barry J. Marhall's review of J. Robin Warren's records on his 25 cases of endoscopic biopsy, many of them showing "mysterious," spiral micro-organisms. The diagnoses in these cases were duodenal ulcer in two, gastric ulcer in seven, gastritis in 12, and "erosions and scars" in four (ref. 1).

The two future Nobel laureates next conducted a prospective study on 100 cases of endoscopy, in which they, as the first researchers ever, came – serendipitously – upon successful cultivation of the mysterious organism, which they named *Helicobacterium pylori*. In the resulting data "there was a strong association between gastritis and the presence of this bacterium. It was found in all patients with duodenal ulcer and 80% of patients with gastric ulcer. In contrast, the presence was rare in patients with non-steroidal drug-related ulcers" (ref. 1).

Then, "Marshall and his colleagues showed that bismuth salts (which had been used to treat gastritis and peptic ulcer disease for many years) killed *H. pylori* in vitro; and, in clinical studies, that bismuth cleared *H. pylori* but the infection would recur unless metronidazole was added to the regimen" (ref. 1).

While the first prospective study's acceptance for publication by *The Lancet* was an exceptionally protracted process – following rejection by the Gastroenterologic Society of Australia – Marshall carried out another type of study as well, very small and very dramatic. "He asked [a colleague] to perform a gastric biopsy on him and then ingested a pure culture of *H. pylori* (10^9 organisms). All was well for 5 days, but then he developed halitosis [bad breath], morning nausea, and recurrent vomiting of acid-free gastric juice. A gastric biopsy on Day 10 showed severe acute gastritis and many *H. pylori*. The symptoms spontaneously resolved after 14 days, ... " (ref. 1).

"This constituted highly suggestive evidence that the organism caused gastritis. But it was far from conclusive, because it involved a single subject and was reported by the very author most wedded to the hypothesis. Thus, replication by others would have been required. Perhaps more important was that the subject, who was none other than Marshall himself, failed to develop an ulcer. Note also that the disease resolved without treatment" (ref. 2).

"What finally convinced doubters of both cause and treatment was something that by its very nature took several years to establish. ... The first trial that was both large enough and rigorous enough to be noticed was conceived by Marshall and Warren in 1984 ... [They] reported that the recurrence rate of duodenal ulcer was much lower in patients whose *H. pylori* were eradicated than in those whose bacteria were not, ... Since the authors were the original proponents of the bacterial hypothesis, moreover, any firm conclusions would first require confirmation by others. This was not ostracism; it was appropriate scientific skepticism" (ref. 2).

While "Marshall and Warren have irrevocably changed clinical practice and have alleviated much human suffering" (ref. 1), they also have made a major contribution to the discipline of etiogenetic epidemiological research: they have, unwittingly, reminded both teachers and students that this research, when successful in its hypothesis generation, and testing of the hypothesis too, is not inherently a matter of competent adherence to established paradigms, or to what used to be termed "the epidemiologic method." Their work is paradigmatic of the potential prowess of extraparadigmatic etiogenetic research.

Chapter 13
From Studies to Knowledge

Abstract Whereas the aim of 'basic' epidemiological research is to provide for the development of products for use in the practice of community medicine, in the population-level counterpart of this the aim is to advance the knowledge-base of the practice.

The population-level research produces *evidence* about (the magnitudes of) the parameters that constitute the objects of any given study, original or derivative; it does not produce *knowledge* about the objects of study. The evidence, is, however, of little value if it does not serve to advance knowledge about the objects of study. The knowledge, to the extent that it is achieved, serves as an input to decisions in the practice; but it does not in itself translate into rational decisions in the practice and, thus, not into guidelines or even recommendations for practice.

Major lines of population-level epidemiological research have, thus far, led to more controversy than knowledge; and where, exceptionally, the need for knowledge has been particularly keenly felt, very elaborate projects of translating evidence into knowledge have been mounted.

For the fact that the accruing evidence does not, by the very nature of science, inherently lead to knowledge relevant to the practice of community medicine there is, we suggest, an identifiable – and removable – cause. We believe it to be the prevailing nature of *medical journalism*. Journals of 'epidemiology' now are not focusing on the concerns of practitioners of community medicine, including updatings of the knowledge-base of this. They play into the common fallacy or conceit that practitioners of medicine are scientists – interested in the continual accrual of evidence and on this basis updating their personal *opinions* about the objects of study.

In the last section of this chapter we outline how epidemiological journalism should be innovated so that there would be a natural progression from epidemiological research to epidemiological knowledge; and in Appendix 3 we outline how this natural process could be supplemented by work in the style of WHO's International Agency for Research on Cancer.

O.S. Miettinen and I. Karp, *Epidemiological Research: An Introduction*,   131
DOI 10.1007/978-94-007-4537-7_13, © Springer Science+Business Media Dordrecht 2012

13.1   Original Study versus Derivative Study

In epidemiological research, studies – pieces of research, research projects (distinct from research programs) – on a given set of objects of study are of two fundamental kinds. An *'original'* study is either the first study on the objects at issue or it is one of this study's replications; and given a set of completed studies on the same set of objects, a *derivative* study is one based on these.

In the *ideal* world of epidemiological research, all of this would be very straightforward. The first one of the original studies would always address a well-designed occurrence relation and have a well-designed methodology to study it; the execution of the methods design would be flawless; and all of this would be replicated with flawless objectivity. The first original study's replications and the reports of these would differ from the first study only in terms of their spatio-temporal particulars and amounts of information (efficiency, size), never in their scientific substance. Replications of the first study would, thus, merely contribute to the available amount of information about (the magnitudes of) the object parameters under study. And at any given stage of the accumulation of the information, a single derivative study would suffice, simply synthesizing the information from all of the completed original studies (as a matter of information – inverse-variance – weighted averaging of the parameters' empirical values from the original studies).

Actual epidemiological research is, still, far from this ideal, in all of the elements in the ideal. Emblematic of this are the prevailing practices in the ultimately relevant, derivative research. In the absence of the availability of a study base for simple synthesis of the results of the entirety of original studies, all well-designed and well-executed, on an expressly defined set of objects of study (for an expressly defined domain of this), 'systematic reviews' draw from the original studies on a given, loosely-defined topic – substituting for a given, expressly-defined object function (for a given domain) – involve the investigators' judgements about the admissibility of particular original studies as inputs into the derivative study; and then, the results are synthesized across varying objects of study (forms of the study result) and methodologies (ultimately as a matter of the design's implementation) – with the synthesis possibly degenerating into mere tallies of 'positive' and 'negative' studies, in disregard of, even, the respective amounts of information (cf. sect. 2.6). Things are even worse: the study base for these reviews generally is seriously selection-/publication-biased (cf. sect. 8.2).

In the needed improvements the beginning naturally would be in the realm of original studies and, in these, in their *objects designs*, for we are, alas, unaware of even a single epidemiological 'systematic review' that could focus on expressly defined, single occurrence relation for an expressly defined domain – the set of studies on this. Equally eminent as a needed improvement is elimination of publication-bias as an engrained feature of epidemiologic-scientific journalism (cf. sect. 13.6).

13.2 The Evidence from a Study

An epidemiological study (on the human level) is a project to produce evidence on (the parameters involved in) an epidemiologically meaningful occurrence relation. The evidence from such a study is imbedded in the *report* from it (along with content of no evidentiary burden, starting from specification of the authors of the report and commonly ending in a 'conclusion'). The reported evidence is either original or derivative in nature (sect. 13.1 above).

An epidemiological study of the original variety can be thought of as a single, unreplicated measurement of the magnitudes of the parameters in the object function of the study; and a derivative study based on a set of original studies can be thought of as making use of replicated measurements on the parameters' values in deriving the best possible single 'reading' on each of them. This is true of hypothesis-testing as well, in which the measurement (multidimensional) is used for discrimination between the null and non-null values of the parameters in the object function.

Evidence about the magnitude of the object of a measurement is first and foremost constituted by the *result* of the measurement, in epidemiological research (on the human level) by the set of *empirical values* of the object parameters from the study (original or derivative). But a critically important added element in the evidence is specification of the *methodology* in the production of the result, as this bears on the result's evidentiary burden through its bearing on the result's (precision and) validity.

In reports on epidemiological research it is always possible – and, hence, necessary – to supplement the object parameters' empirical values with *measures of imprecision* of these ('standard errors' or 'confidence intervals'). These are a reflection of the study's degree of informativeness (about the parameters' values), determined by the study's efficiency together with its size. They thus represent not the study's results per se but one of the two important qualities of these.

For a study result's degree of *bias* – lack of validity – no measure can be derived from the study; if it could, the corresponding requisite correction would be made in the result. The degree of bias in the result remains a matter of judgement, by whoever is concerned with the result from the study – the 'systematic review' investigators in the context of any original study, and the relevant scientific community as for a derivative study.

13.3 Interpretation of the Evidence

Evidence from an epidemiological study is, as just set forth, imbedded in the report from the study; and specifically it is, so we implied, constituted by words and numbers describing the study's results on the magnitudes of the parameters in the designed object of the study, these together with description of the genesis of these results, verbal and numerical description of this too, augmented by measures of the consequent imprecisions of the parameters' empirical values.

Interpretation of this evidence we take to be formation of a view of what this reporting of the evidence actually means, what the thus-communicated evidence actually is. We thus sharply distinguish between interpretation of evidence, in this meaning of it, and inference from the evidence (sect. 13.4 below).

In the context of the present level of development of the shared concepts and terms among epidemiological researchers, the interpretation of the report of, and hence the evidence from, epidemiological studies can be challenging, insofar as avoidance of misunderstanding is the concern (sect. 2.6). To the extent that this is the case, it is a serious problem. For, "Where concepts are firm, clear and generally accepted, and the methods of reasoning and arriving at conclusion are agreed between men (at least the majority of those who have anything to do with these matters), there and only there is it possible to construct a science, formal or empirical." So wrote Isaiah Berlin in his venerable *The Proper Study of Mankind: An Anthology of Essays* (Hardy H, Hansheer R, Editors; 1997; p. 61).

Emblematic about the status quo are some central routines in epidemiological study reports at present. There still eminently is 'cohort study' and 'case-control study,' rather than merely *the* etiologic/etiogenetic study (sect. 6.5). And even though these two are thought of as alternatives to each other, reported from the former usually is a result in terms of 'relative risk,' with 'odds ratio' the common counterpart of this from the latter (sect. 2.6) – both of these terms properly referring to a parameter rather than the result of a study (which in the context of an etiologic/etiogenetic study generally is the ratio of two empirical rates, two incidence densities). 'Significantly increased risk' in the determinant's index category is a common expression for the strictly particularistic fact that the rate in the study experience was higher in this category, and that the difference was statistically (*sic*) significant – the actual risk implications of this, if any, being a matter not of experience per se but inference from it (sect. 13.4 below). Just as unobservable/undocumentable as causal increase in risk or rate is, of course, 'reduction' (inherently causal) in it, also commonly reported as a purported result of an epidemiological study (sect. 2.6). Neither one of them can be 'found' in, or 'shown' by, an epidemiological study.

Particularly great challenges of interpretation are exemplified in Appendix 2.

13.4 Inference from the Evidence

An epidemiological researcher, and any consumer of the research likewise, faces a profound yet unavoidable limitation of the studies, derivative ones included. However well-designed be the object function of the study and however good the design of the study's methodology as well as execution of this, the inescapable problem is, for a start, that the object of study has an *abstract* – placeless and timeless – domain as its referent, while the study result inherently has a *particularistic* referent (i.e., the study base, spatio-temporally specific). This constitutes a notable challenge for learning about descriptive – acausal, purely phenomenal – objects of study already.

The challenge is greater yet when the object of study is *causal* – noumenal in this sense – and the study proper is, as is commonplace, *non-experimental* – and subject to *biases* even in descriptive terms.

Thus, however correct may be someone's interpretation of the evidence from a study (as to what the report from the study means in this respect; sect. 13.3 above), his/her *inference* about the object of study in the light of the evidence remains a matter of subjective judgements, leading only to his/her personal *opinion* about the abstract truth in question.

13.5   Knowledge from the Evidence

Scientific research, epidemiological like any other, is a quest for scientific *knowledge* – for presumably truthful insights into the abstract.

Whereas evidence from epidemiological research on any given object of inquiry provides for only personal opinions about the truth at issue (sect. 13.4 above), the challenge that immediately results from this is reasonable conceptualization of the nature, the essence, of epidemiological knowledge. And with this resolved, it remains to understand how the evidence on any given object of desired, epidemiological knowledge can be translated into that knowledge. These challenges have remained too little addressed and incompletely resolved, with the consequence that epidemiological knowledge, even on obviously important topics, still tends to remain ill-defined or controversial (ch. 2).

Pre-scientifically it used to be known – firmly, for a very long time – that disease commonly is a matter of aberrant distribution among the four 'humors' in the body. It also was known that 'miasma' – vapors emanating from the soil, swamps, and decaying organic matter – are causal to disease, and that disease can be alleviated (or perhaps even cured) by blood-letting.

In this modern era of health science it has just recently become known, from epidemiological research, that dietary fats are causal to cardiovascular disease, while research previously had persuaded experts that it was dietary carbohydrates that had this effect; and the latter may get to be the knowledge in the future as well (sect. 2.1).

Epidemiological knowledge, even in this era of epidemiological science (in the research meaning of this), is not inherently true; it is, even, subject to being a denial of previous scientific knowledge – science being, by its nature, self-corrective rather than simply ('linearly') progressive. It is, first-off, knowledge in the sense of experts (in the relevant scientific community) having come to a more-or-less common, *shared belief* about the truth at issue. These experts can defend their shared belief; their knowledge is *active* in this sense.

Secondarily, there is others' knowledge about the experts' shared belief, *passive* knowledge in this sense, knowledge that cannot be justified by those who possess it. Most people know that dietary fats are causal to cardiovascular disease, but only experts on the subject can justify this belief (with the justification subject to being mistaken).

The public-health authorities of Denmark, in 2011, adopted a public policy consequent to their second-hand knowledge – secondary to first-hand, expert knowledge – about the health consequence of fats in the diet. They introduced a tax on purchases of foods high in saturated fats. This policy may well be ill-founded and even counterproductive: the result may well be, for one, an epidemic of obesity in Denmark, just as there already is in the fats-averse U.S., for example.

Express formulation of expert knowledge on matters epidemiological has not been prone to emerge spontaneously in the relevant scientific community; it has required deliberations and formulations and by topic-specific *expert committees*. But this, too, has been problematic, as that which emerges is prone to be dependent on which set of experts constitutes the committee, among other factors.

Spontaneous movement from evidence to knowledge within the relevant scientific communities could be, so we believe, substantially enhanced by suitable innovations in medical journalism (sect. 13.6 below); and related to this, the culture of 'task forces' on preventive healthcare could – and should – be substantially improved (Apps. 1, 2, 3).

Two examples of express efforts to derive knowledge from the evidence produced by epidemiological research (incl. 'bench' research; sect. 1.2) are particularly instructive: the work on the *Smoking and Health* report (1964) of an ad-hoc advisory committee to the Surgeon General of the Public Health Service of the U.S. Department of Health, Education, and Welfare; and the work on the continually accruing *IARC Monographs on the Evaluation of Carcinogenic Risks in Humans*, IARC being the International Agency for Research on Cancer within the World Health Organization.

The smoking-and-health committee received from the National Library of Medicine a total of 1,100 articles (p. 14). "In addition to the special reports prepared under contracts, many conferences, seminar-like meetings, consultations, visits and correspondence made available to the Committee a large amount of material and a considerable amount of well-informed and well-reasoned opinion and advice" (p. 15).

"There were an uncounted number of meetings of subcommittees and other lesser gatherings. Between November 1962 and December 1963, the full Committee held nine sessions each lasting from two to four days" (p. 15).

"All members of the Committee were schooled in the high standards and criteria implicit in making scientific assessments; if any member lacked even a small part of such schooling he received it in good measure from the strenuous debates that took place at consultations and at meetings at the subcommittees and the whole Committee" (p. 19).

"It is advisable, however, to discuss briefly certain criteria which, although applicable to all judgements involved in this Report, are especially significant for judgements based upon *the epidemiologic method* ... When coupled with the other data, results from epidemiologic studies can provide the basis on which judgements of causality can be made" (pp. 19–20; italics ours).

"In carrying out studies through the use of this epidemiologic method, many factors, variables, and results of investigations must be considered to determine first whether an association actually exists between an attribute or agent and a disease. ... If it be shown that an association exists, then the question is asked: 'Does the association have a causal significance?'" (p. 20).

"To judge or evaluate the causal significance of the association ... a number of criteria must be utilized, no one of which is an all-sufficient basis for judgement. These criteria include:

(a) The consistency of the association
(b) The strength of the association
(c) The specificity of the association
(d) The temporal relationship of the association
(e) The coherence of the association

These criteria were used in various sections of this Report. the most extensive and illuminating account of their utilization is found in chapter 9 in the section entitled 'Evaluation of the Association Between Smoking and Lung Cancer'" (p. 20).

The application of these criteria led to these Conclusions in respect to lung cancer (p. 196):

1. Cigarette smoking is causally related to lung cancer in men. ... The data for women, though less extensive, point to the same direction.
2. The risk of developing lung cancer increases with duration of smoking and the number of cigarettes smoked per day, and it is diminished by discontinuing smoking.
3. The risk of developing cancer of the lung for the combined group of pipe smokers, cigar smokers, and pipe and cigar smokers is greater than in non-smokers, but much less than for cigarette smokers. The data are insufficient to warrant a conclusion for each group individually.

Three remarks may be called for here. First, at the time of this Report, epidemiology was commonly defined as research by means of "the epidemiologic method" (cf. above), and its principal types were termed, as in this Report, "prospective study" and "retrospective study" (which later got to be termed cohort study and case-control study, respectively).

Second, the "criteria" for causal inference deployed by the Committee were the "considerations" famously elaborated by the statistician A.B. Hill the year after the Report's publication. (He was not a member of the 10-member Committee; its statistician was W.G. Cochran.) But *those criteria/considerations are largely untenable*. To wit, the strength of a non-causal association can be very strong, as in the case between match-consumption and lung cancer, for example; and this association exhibits a strong dose-response pattern – a topic under "Coherence of association" (p. 123).

Third, curiously missing from the "criteria" is the *biological plausibility of the association's causality*, which Hill included, and the *plausibility of confounding as an explanation* of the association, which Hill did not include. The section immediately in front of Conclusions is entitled "Other Etiologic Factors and Confounding Variables" (p. 183 ff), but it simply expands on the point that "a causal hypothesis for the cigarette-smoking-lung cancer relationship does not exclude other factors" (p. 193). The ones addressed are "Occupational Hazards," "Urbanization, Industrialization, and Air Pollution," "Previous Respiratory Infection," and "Other Factors." There is no word about any of these – or any other confounders – as possible explanations of the association between smoking and lung cancer.

As for the *IARC Monographs*, their Preamble – http://monographs.iarc.fr/ENG/ Preamble/CurrentPreamble.pdf – is instructive reading. "The Preamble is primarily a statement of scientific principles, rather than specification of working procedures" (p. 1). It deserves to be quite extensively quoted here.

In these monographs, the potentially carcinogenic "agents" are viewed in very inclusive terms: "specific chemicals, groups of related chemicals, complex mixtures, occupational and environmental exposures, cultural and behavioural practices, biological organisms and physical agents. This list of categories may expand as causation of, and susceptibility to, malignant disease become more fully understood" (p. 2).

"Although the Monographs have emphasized hazard identification [a hazard being "an agent that is capable of causing cancer under some circumstances"], important issues may also involve dose-response assessment. In many cases, the same epidemiological and experimental data used to evaluate a cancer hazard can also be used to estimate a dose-response relationship" (pp. 2–3).

"The *Monographs* are used by national and international authorities to make risk assessments, formulate decisions concerning preventive measures, provide effective cancer control programs and decide among alternative options for public health decisions. ... These evaluations represent only one part of the body of information on which public health decisions may be based. ... Therefore, no recommendation is given with regard to regulation or legislation, which are the responsibility of individual governments or other international organizations" (p. 3).

"Working Group Members generally have published significant research related to the carcinogenicity of the agents being reviewed, and IARC uses literature searches to identify most experts. Working Group Members are selected on the basis of (a) knowledge and experience and (b) absence of real or apparent conflicts of interests. Consideration may also be given to demographic diversity and balance of scientific findings and views" (p. 4).

"Approximately one year in advance of the meeting of a Working Group, the agents to be reviewed are announced on the *Monographs* programme website (http:// monographs.iarc.fr) and participants are selected by IARC staff in consultation with other experts. Subsequently, relevant biological and epidemiological data are

collected by IARC from recognized sources of information on carcinogenesis, ...
Meeting participants who are asked to prepare preliminary working papers for
specific sections are expected to supplement the IARC literature searches with their
own searches. ... The working papers are compiled by IARC staff and sent, prior
to the meeting, to Working Group Members and Invited Specialists for review. The
Working Group meets at IARC for seven to eight days to discuss and finalize the
texts and to formulate the evaluations. ... Care is taken to ensure that each study
summary is written or reviewed by someone not associated with the study being
considered. ... IARC Working Groups strive to achieve a consensus evaluation"
(pp. 5–6).

"Several types of epidemiological study contribute to the assessment of carcinogenicity in humans – cohort studies, case-control studies, correlation (ecological)
studies, and intervention studies. Rarely, results from randomized trials may be
available. Case reports and case series of cancer in humans may also be reviewed. ... In correlation studies, individual exposure is not documented, which
renders this type of study more prone to confounding. In some circumstances,
however, correlation studies may be more informative than analytical study designs"
(pp. 8–9).

"It is necessary to take into account the possible roles of bias, confounding and
chance in the interpretation of epidemiological studies. ... Potential confounding
... should have been dealt with either in the design of the study, such as by
matching, or via the analysis, by statistical adjustment. In cohort studies [our semi-
cohort studies; sect. 6.4], comparison with local rates of disease may or may not
be more appropriate than those with national rates. ... Detailed analyses of both
relative and absolute risks in relation to temporal variables, such as age at first
exposure, time since first exposure, duration of exposure, cumulative exposure, peak
exposure (when appropriate) and time since cessation of exposure, are reviewed
and summarized when available. Analyses of temporal relationships may be useful
in making causal inferences. ... After the quality of individual epidemiological
studies of cancer has been summarized and assessed, a judgement is made of the
strength of evidence that the agent in question is carcinogenic to humans. In making
its judgements, the Working Group considers several criteria for causality (Hill
1965). A strong association (e.g., a large relative risk) is more likely to indicate
causality than a weak association, ... If the risk increases with exposure, this is
considered a strong indication of causality, ... " (pp. 9–11).

Upon the review of evidence also from experimental animals as well as "mechanistic and other relevant data" (p. 15), "the body of evidence is considered as a
whole, in order to reach an overall evaluation of the carcinogenicity of the agent in
humans. ... The categorization of the agent is a matter of scientific judgement
that reflects the strength of the evidence derived from studies in humans and
in experimental animals and from mechanistic and other relevant data" (p. 22).
The categories are: "Group 1: The agent is *carcinogenic to humans* ... Group
4: The agent is *probably not carcinogenic to humans*" (pp. 22-3; italics in the
original).

Looking back at these excerpts from the Preamble to the IARC Monographs, the points of instructive note include these:

1. Whereas we think of carcinogenic factors in the categories of constitutional, environmental, and behavioral, IARC's classification of carcinogenic "agents" is quite different from this. Those "specific chemicals, groups of related chemicals, complex mixtures" are, to us, potential carcinogenic factors only when they are constituents (acquired) of a person's constitution, or subject to becoming constitutional on account of a person's behavior or environment; "occupational" factors are, to us, either behavioral or (micro-)environmental; "exposures" are, to us, all environmental (even if as a result of behavior); "behavioural practices" are not, to us, alternatives to "cultural" ones but, potentially, cultural in their origin; all "organisms" are, to us, "biomedical"; all carcinogenetic "agents" are, to us, chemical, physical, or biological, involved in the constitutional, behavioral, or environmental carcinogenic factors (such as inflammation, smoking, and air pollution); and "causation" is, to us, that which a cause may bring about, depending on "susceptibility" to the cause, without the latter being a carcinogen (while sunlight is a carcinogen, albinism is a related susceptibility factor but not a carcinogen).

2. IARC distinguishes between "epidemiological and experimental data," implying that epidemiological data inherently are non-experimental. To us, research data are epidemiological if the intent in their production was to advance the practice of community medicine, with the research quite possibly experimental, including in the laboratory (sect. 1.2).

3. IARC is concerned not only with identification of carcinogenic hazards but also with quantification of carcinogenic effects – "dose-response assessment." The Monographs have "emphasized" the former, understandably, as epidemiological research has tended not to get past hypothesis testing (ch. 2).

4. IARC sees itself in the service of public-health authorities in their decisions about preventive-oncologic measures, but: *no recommendation is given.*" This is in sharp contrast with what is done by the Canadian Task Force on Preventive Health Care and by the Preventive Medicine Task Force in the U.S.; and we think that the IARC is right on this important matter. See Appendices 1 and 2.

5. IARC has a very elaborate scheme of assuring the greatest possible validity of its Conclusions, which again is instructive of how major is the transition from evidence to knowledge, seen to result only from experts' "consensus evaluation" of the evidence. As the Working Groups have to "strive to achieve" consensus, the question is, How concordant would tend to be the conclusions of two or more similarly constituted and similarly working expert groups, addressing the same question.

6. IARC reflects our contemporary normal-science conception of "types of epidemiological study" on humans. Exceptionally, though, it prefers to use "correlation study" as the term for what now is commonly known as ecological study. The preference is curious, as the adjective is no more apt a descriptor of studies with populations as the units of observation than studies of the

other type – notably "cohort studies" and "case–control studies" – which IARC characterizes as representing "analytical study designs," in unjustifiable deference to epidemiological tradition. (Those studies are not about analysis, and the logic in them is synthetic rather than analytic.)

7. IARC seems to use "interpretation" as a synonym for "evaluation" in judgements about epidemiological evidence, while for us interpretation is a challenge in understanding the meaning of the report of a study (as to what the result actually was, and how it actually came about, according to the report; sect. 13.3). But we are fully comfortable with the idea that a study needs to be judged in respect to "the possible role of bias [descriptive], confounding and chance" (sect. 8.2).

8. Different from IARC, we've left behind the common idea that "Potential confounding … should have been dealt with either in the design of the study, such as by matching, or in the analysis, by statistical adjustment." We now think of study design as specifying everything that will intentionally go into the genesis of the study result, including the statistical model and its fitting to the data; and confounding is "dealt with" in the design stage of that model in non-experimental etiogenetic research and, thereby, in the synthesis (*sic*) of the study data (into the study result and measures of its precision), without the latter being an alternative to the former (chs. 7, 8). Matching generally is a matter of the sampling for the base series being discriminate/stratified (according to the distribution of the case series). This stratification needs to be accounted for in the model; but it is this modeling, and not the matching, that constitutes control of confounding. (That modeling achieves the control even in the absence of the matching.)

9. IARC evidently takes, quite exceptionally, the concept of cohort study to encompass what we here term semi-cohort study (sect. 6.4); and despite the primitive nature of this kind of study, IARC, surprisingly to us, seems to take it as potentially providing quite meaningful evidence about oncogenesis. We think that the 'healthy worker effect' is symptomatic of unhealthy study. (There is no 'sick patient effect' in clinical research.)

10. IARC conducts "detailed analyses" in respect to "temporal variables" in terms that are different from what we consider appropriate. Evidently in reference to histories in etiogenetic studies, these IARC concerns include "age at first exposure, time since first exposure, duration of exposure, cumulative exposure," etc., with the idea that "analysis of temporal relationships may be useful in making causal inferences." Instead of any of these, our concern is the study's objects design in respect to the index and reference histories on the scale of etiogenetic time, across the entire relevant range of this, with the index-reference contrasts based on these.

11. Based on the human evidence, "a judgement is made of the strength of [this] evidence that the agent in question is carcinogenic to humans" – as though the concern always were with qualitative inference (cf. # 3 above). And in this, the Working Groups are said to deploy the "several criteria of causality" enunciated

(as "considerations") but A.B. Hill – despite the obvious untenability of many of these (cf. the Smoking and Health example above).

12. The Conclusions, representing the knowledge formulated by any given Working Group, like those assessments/evaluations of the evidence from the studies, also are only qualitative in nature (cf. # 11 above, in contrast to # 3). Yet, only quantitative knowledge is the appropriate basis for authorities to set 'threshold limit values,' for example (cf. # 3 and # 4 above).

13.6   The Needed Innovations

The prime example of the fruits of twentieth-century epidemiological research is, arguably at least, the attained knowledge about the health effects – adverse, on risk of lung cancer most notably – of smoking, cigarette smoking in particular. The research effort was huge (sect. 2.7) and its translation into 'official' knowledge very elaborate (sect. 13.5 above).

Even more elaborate have been and are the periodic processes of translating into knowledge the available evidence concerning possible carcinogenesis, the way they are performed by the International Agency for Research on Cancer for the production of the *IARC Monographs* (sect. 13.5 above). Might it be that awe of these efforts at the definition of epidemiological knowledge is at the root of the *Epidemiologic Reviews* typically addressing epidemiological studies rather than the knowledge derived from these? (sect. 2.6.)

Very respectable about the IARC (of the WHO) is its heeding of the principle that relevant scientific knowledge is to be seen to be only one category of the relevant inputs into rational decisions in public-health practice. IARC understands that *evidence, or even knowledge from it, does not translate into justifiable recommendations about decisions in practice*, in disregard of all other relevant considerations, generally peculiar to the particular contexts of the decisions (sect. 13.5). This point is compellingly argued by R.A. Pielke, Jr. in his *The Honest Broker: Making Sense of Science in Policy and Politics* (2007).

This feature of the IARC reviews, which merely is what one should expect, gains its poignancy from its unwitting foils, from the various 'official' producers of *'evidence-based' guidelines/recommendations* for public-health policy about preventive medicine. Particularly notable as such foils of the IARC are the Canadian Task Force on Preventive Health Care (App. 1) and the Preventive Medicine Task Force in the U.S., both programmatically producing recommendations/guidelines for decisions in the practice of what they take to be preventive medicine. And notable about these particular programs of recommendations-production is not merely that this is what they do but also the level of seriousness of the work as for what types of panel of people does it and how (Apps. 1, 2) – how casual all of this is, in contrast to the work of the IARC.

Those task forces produce policy recommendations most eminently in respect to various types of *screening* for a cancer, which has become a common concern of epidemiological researchers and hence a concern also in the *Epidemiologic Reviews* when a particular cancer is addressed (2001 issue) and even as such (2011 issue; sect. 2.6). This interest of epidemiologists in screening for a cancer as a purported topic in community-level preventive medicine is an outgrowth of past programs of mobile units of fluoroscopic screening for pulmonary tuberculosis, such case-finding as an element in the prevention of the spread of the infection in the community. In Japan there now are public-health programs of screening for lung cancer as direct, seamless outgrowths of previous programs of screening for tuberculosis. But cancer, different from tuberculosis, is not a communicable disease, so that its detection and treatment in no way serves prevention of the spread of the disease in the community.

So determined are those task forces in their production of recommendations on – for or against – screenings for cancers (and other diseases too), based on the mistaken idea that screening for an illness is a preventive intervention; so misguided consequently is the common idea among epidemiologists as for the nature of the research and knowledge needed for public policies for or against the screenings (public funding of the initial tests in these); and so different are the genuine – clinical – counterparts of these, that we deal with the topic quite extensively (sects. 2.6, 7.2; ch. 11; App. 2), even though at issue is not epidemiological – but meta-epidemiological clinical – research.

As translation of the evidence from epidemiological research into knowledge for public-health practice is commonly absent (sect. 2.6), occasionally very elaborately done (sect. 13.5 above), and in yet other instances done very flippantly but used as the practically sole basis of guidelines/recommendations regarding practice (Apps. 1, 2), *something is fundamentally amiss in the evidence-to-knowledge phase of the genesis of epidemiological knowledge*, serving to sustain various anomalies also in the production of the evidence – the single most notable example of the latter being the research on screening for a cancer.

The fundamental anomaly is, we suggest, near-complete absence of that which, in science, normally would produce those evidence-to-knowledge transmutations, namely: *public discourse* among the members of the relevant scientific communities. This anomaly is rooted in *the prevailing general culture of our medical journals*, which do not serve as open forums for this critically important element in the normal process by which empirical science progresses. Today these journals are mainly directed to practicing physicians, to whom they supply fresh evidence – and 'conclusions' based solely on this! – instead of what doctors actually need from science, namely updated knowledge.

A distinction should be made between journals of *medicine* – for practitioners of it – and those of *medical science* – for medical scientists; and in the latter there is a need to distinguish between journals of *evidence* and those of *inference* (from evidence; sect. 13.4). Genuine journals of medical science would not merely freely allow, but would actually encourage and invite, public discourse among scientists. This would be so in respect to inference in particular, as it is public discourse about this, by the very nature of science, that has the capacity to converge into experts' shared belief, into genuine knowledge on a topic in medical (as in any other) science; and difficulties in this would also serve to underscore the deficiencies in the available evidence, inviting remedies for them.

As for quintessentially applied epidemiological – and meta-epidemiological clinical – science specifically, a third kind of needed medical journalism concerns its *theory* – concepts and terminology for a start (Preface) and then principles (sect. 1.3). This, too, is less than satisfactory at present, in that consensus-seeking public discourse is missing in this area as well. And so it still is that textbooks of epidemiological research generally are mainly about study of the etiology/etiogenesis of 'disease' rather than illness (disease/defect/injury or *morbus/vitium/trauma*); addressed is methodology of the research in total disregard of the studies' objects design; and in the studies themselves a major distinction still is routinely made between 'cohort' and 'case-control' studies instead of proceeding from each of these into the corresponding corrected conceptions, into that which is essential in all etiologic/etiogenetic studies in this genre of them (chs. 5, 6). As another major example, the textbooks still are prone not to make the profound distinction between inquiries that are epidemiological research and ones that are part of epidemiological practice (sect. 14.1).

More on the needed innovations in the translation of evidence into knowledge for the practice of community medicine is given in Appendix 3.

As for the evidence itself in specifically epidemiologic journals, its *publication bias* remains a serious problem; but this too is remediable: Reporting on population-level epidemiological studies should be accepted for publication before any results are at hand – that is, upon the authors having completed the Introduction, Objects Design, and Methods Design sections of the report and the sections having passed peer review as well as review by the journal's editorial board. No report should be accepted belatedly, after the study plan's implementation has already begun. Each timely acceptance of the study plan for ultimate publication of the report should be a matter of accessible record (incl. for the purposes of grant applications and their peer reviews, in addition to the needs of derivative studies).

That early acceptance of the ultimate report on a study would not mean that whatever gets to be written in it under Results and Discussion – and in the Summary/Abstract – has advance approval for publication. The journal's editorial board has the responsibility (to the scientific community) to make sure that the writing accords with the principles of this. Prime among these is the imperative to clearly and correctly distinguish between particularistic facts about study results and inferential ideas based on these. As for this, pervasive still is writing about study results as though causality (or lack of it) had been observed and documented in a study (cf. sect. 4.2). Quotes in this text illustrate this misleading writing, starting in section 2.2 ("showed no reduction in," "did not affect").

With these innovations, epidemiologic journals would much better focus on genuine contributions to evidence, minimizing obfuscating 'litter-ature.' "I coined the term 'litter-ature' to denote that too much of the medical literature is littered with misleading and false-positive findings," writes Eric Topol in his *The Creative Destruction of Medicine: How the Digital Revolution Will Create Better Health Care* (2012; pp. 31-2).

We add that even more influential as a source of publication bias generally is the common opposite: 'cleaning' out of the literature reports with 'negative' results, commonly meaning only relatively imprecise results, however valid.

Chapter 14
Fact-finding in Epidemiological Practice

Abstract Practice of community medicine involves, quite centrally, acquisition of statistics (frequency numbers) on the cared-for population and making, on this basis, inferences about frequencies of health hazards and illnesses (levels of morbidity) in the population. The epitome of this is the 'investigation' of an epidemic with a view to inferences about it, descriptive for one and etiogenetic for another – this as the basis of controlling the epidemic's extent and prevention of its recurrence. Commonly involved are sample surveys and their sample-to-population inferences – something termed 'survey research' by statisticians. *There thus is a strong tendency to suffer the delusion that practice of community medicine is science.*

In this chapter we first outline the profound difference between fact-finding in epidemiological practice and that in (population-level) epidemiological research, supplementing this with description of fact-finding in the epidemiological practice of the public-health agency of Canada's capital city.

We then describe fact-finding in a very different line of public-health practice in Ottawa. Now that national health insurance has been introduced into Canada, *clinical* medicine in this country is public healthcare, with its administration a provincial responsibility. The main concerns of the provincial ministers of health now are *quality assurance* and *cost containment* of clinical medicine, hospital-based care in particular. We describe what fact-finding in this vein the Ontario government now obligates to the hospitals in the province, and how Ottawa hospitals are responding to these.

Finally, given the centrally important place of quality assurance – economic as well as medical quality – of clinical care, and of hospital-based care in particular, at present and ever-increasingly in the future, we devote considerable attention to how this quality assurance could be substantially improved – by future practitioners of epidemiology.

14.1   Fact-finding vis-à-vis Research

Fact-finding is not what a piece of epidemiological research is about. For, the researchers are not concerned with the assembled facts per se, not individually nor in the aggregate, not out of interest nor as a basis for action on the individuals or the population contributing to the study base. Even the study result – this aggregate fact on the study base – is but a window – barely transparent – into what a piece of epidemiological research really is about: an abstract truth rather than anything particularistically factual. If the truth at issue about the abstract be known, facts about whatever population-time or whatever series of person-moments would be irrelevant from the vantage of epidemiological research.

In epidemiological *practice*, by contrast, an epidemiological 'study' (*sic*) is a project of fact-finding. In it, the concern is to establish a fact, or a set of these, about the cared-for population, relevant to the care for this population. Paradigmatic about this is study in the meaning of *investigation of an epidemic* as to its pattern and degree of spread and, especially, as to its etiogenesis. The findings from this investigation are not results for publication in a scientific journal. They are, instead, inputs into ad-hoc decisions about control of the epidemic at issue and about future prevention of other similar epidemics in the cared-for population (sect. 14.4).

This chapter is devoted to delineation of fact-finding in epidemiological practice, with two aims: to illustrate the distinction between this and epidemiological research, and to help make more concrete the concept of epidemiology as practice of community medicine (sect. 1.1) – the advancement of which is the raison d'être of epidemiology in the research meaning of the term (sect. 1.2).

The last section this chapter we regard as being particularly important in respect to *modern public health*, in which quality assurance and cost containment of *clinical* care are the central concerns, and in which epidemiologists can make a critically important contribution to society.

14.2   Fact-finding by Use of Routine Sources

In fact-finding about the population's demographic composition, and state of health, a community doctor can make use of data readily available from routine sources. Thus, Ottawa Public Health can ascertain the city population's demographics from the Provincial Health Planning Database (maintained by the Ontario Ministry of Health and Long-term Care) and from *Ottawa Facts and Research* and *Ottawa Facts, Data Handbook* (produced by the City of Ottawa); its overall rates of mortality and hospitalization, as well as rates of mortality specific to leading causes of death and hospitalization rates specific for age and gender, from the Provincial Health Planning Database; its rates of morbidity and mortality from any given cancer, specific for age and gender, from the Ontario Cancer Registry (maintained by

Cancer Care Ontario) and the Provincial Health Planning Database. The Provincial Health Planning Database contains information also on rates of injuries, poisonings, suicide, etc.

Besides, Ottawa Public Health can obtain the information on the rates of communicable-diseases morbidity from the Integrated Public Health System of the Ontario Ministry of Health and Long-term Care.

14.3   Fact-finding by Ad-hoc Surveys and Monitorings

Fact-finding by the use of routine sources a community doctor commonly supplements with data from ad-hoc surveys and monitorings, conducted by the doctor's agency (possibly commissioning for this purpose another agency or organization) or by another agency or organization independently of the community doctor's agency.

The City of Ottawa 2006 Health Status Report gives several examples of these. As one example, it "surveyed 800 mothers of 3 [sic] and 6-month-old infants to determine health status, factors influencing health and the utilization of health care services by parents of infants. The survey also identified trends of methods parents used to care for their infants" (p. 133). Another example is the Rapid Risk Factor Surveillance System, conducted by the Institute for Social Research, York University, on behalf of Ottawa Public Health. It is "an ongoing random-digit-dialed telephone survey of adults aged 18 years and over, … The first wave of data collection for Ottawa began in April 2001. Households are randomly selected from all households in the City of Ottawa and a sample of 100 residents are surveyed every month regarding health risk behaviours, knowledge, attitudes, and awareness about health related topics of importance to public health such as smoking, immunization, sun safety etc" (p. 134).

An example of extrinsic "survey" is the Canadian Community Health Survey (CCHS), conducted by Statistics Canada, data from which are available from the Ontario Ministry of Health and Long-term Care. "This is a national population household survey for all provinces and territories in Canada … . The survey collects information on the health of the Canadian population aged 12 and older as well as socio-economic data. The survey runs in a two-year collection cycle and is comprised of two distinct parts: a health region-level survey in the first year with a total sample of 130,000 and a provincial-level survey in the second year with a total sample of 30,000. Data collection commenced in 2000. A broad range of topics are examined in the survey on health status, determinants of health and health system utilization. Data available for Ottawa includes 2000-01 and 2003, and the sample size is approximately 1900. The CCHS is the data source for many of the Health Indicators generated by Statistics Canada and the Canadian Institute for Health Information" (p. 133).

A program of successive, periodic surveys on the same topics on the same, sampled population we think of as being a program of *monitoring* (over time) rather than a survey (at a particular time).

14.4 Investigations of Epidemics

Even if endemic morbidity from non-communicable, 'chronic' diseases has become
a major concern in the practice of epidemiology, community diagnoses about
epidemics of communicable disease and control of these remains an important
component in this practice. As described in the City of Ottawa 2006 Health Status
Report, "Ottawa Public Health investigates all potential respiratory outbreaks in
long-term care residences, hospitals, day care centres, schools and other institutions.
Investigations also occur for potential outbreaks reported from the community or
those detected by routine communicable disease surveillance. Outbreak investigations can include case-finding, contact tracing, infection control, risk assessment,
and immunization. ... In 2004, there were 196 confirmed outbreaks in the City
of Ottawa. ... There were 62 outbreaks related to respiratory infections and
134 outbreaks related to enteric infections" (p. 111).

14.5 Quality Assessment of Hospital Care

Epidemiological practice of healthcare in the meaning of community-level preventive medicine (sect. 1.1) – informed by fact-findings that are an integral part of it
(sects. 14.2, 14.3, 14.4 above) as supplements to inputs from general epidemiological knowledge (ch. 2; sect. 13.5) – used to be the entirety of epidemiological
practice. This was the case when the domain of *public health* was coterminous with
that of *community health* in reference to professional healthcare (paramedical as
well as medical), when public health thus was extrinsic to the domain of clinical
healthcare. In this framework, epidemiological practice was expressly *societal*
healthcare, not only societally financed but also governed by public policies, while
clinical practice was essentially private and autonomous, essentially outside societal
concerns.

   All of this was upended by the advent of national health insurance, initially in the
U.K. in 1848, followed by other countries, Canada included. In the U.S., outside the
Veterans' Administration, it still is limited to Medicare for the elderly and Medicaid
for the indigent. *National health insurance brought clinical medicine into the domain
of public health*. As a consequence, clinical medicine became the greater segment
of public-health medicine, by far, relative to community medicine.

   While the aggregate cost of healthcare in a modern society already consumes
a huge proportion of the Gross Domestic Product, this cost is growing at a rate
that unquestionably is unsustainable. With a view to clinical medicine in particular,
the central mantra of modern public health – and today's Minister of Health –
thus is *cost containment*; and as the pursuit of this may compromise the quality
of healthcare, *quality assurance* has become an associated, added mantra.

   Promulgators of public-health *policy* have adduced various schemes of pursuing
the hoped-for cost-containment in healthcare, including, in Canada, restrictions in

numbers of doctors in particular disciplines of medicine. But an unintended consequence has commonly been a reduction in individuals' access to justifiable care.

Practicing *epidemiologists*, as public-health officials, are accustomed to monitoring health-related goings-on (sect. 14.3) and taking or recommending remedial
action when called for in the interest of public health. They could, very usefully,
bring this culture to clinical medicine, perhaps to hospitals first and foremost, where
half of the healthcare expenditure is incurred in countries like Canada.

They could – and really should – introduce continual, sampling-based *monitoring
of the care processes* (rather than outcomes) into hospitals within a given jurisdiction. This would be a matter of retrospectively documenting (by records abstraction)
the care for individual patients throughout their sojourns in a given type of hospital.
The case-specific findings would be submitted for review by a suitable panel of
experts, for them to *identify lapses of quality, economic and/or medical*, in the
care. An elementary and cardinal lack of requisite quality is, of course, lack of the
requisite recordings for use in this monitoring (i.a.).

Reports of the untoward findings – of the *rates* of these – would be submitted to
the appropriate administrators, for possible remedial action (or laudation).

While science is supposed to be self-corrective, medicine is supposed to be self-
policing. The essence of self-policing in medicine is active and competent pursuit
of identification of physicians' substandard behaviors and, upon their identification,
bringing these to the attention of the relevant officials for remedial – or punitive –
action. As we outlined above, practicing epidemiologists, when in the service of
modern public health, are uniquely qualified to do this in respect to clinical care;
and so: *noblesse oblige*.

Given that good healthcare is not only medically but also economically good – not
only effective but *cost-effective* as well – and given also the ever-deepening cost
crisis in modern, societally sponsored healthcare – in modern *public health*, that
is – the topic of quality assurance in clinical healthcare deserves more deliberate
consideration here than the little sketch above, ultimately with a view to the
role(s) we think practicing epidemiologists need to adopt – as genuine 'clinical
epidemiologists,' without the term being self-contradictory.

With screening for a cancer now a misguided exception (Apps. 1, 2), clinical
medicine has retained a good deal of autonomy within the society even after
the advent of national health insurance. Societies regulate industries as for the
marketing of medications and medical devices, but they still refrain from regulation
of the use of these products – or other professional actions – by clinicians.

Regarding the autonomous quality-assurance in clinical medicine, M.S. Liang
and P. Fortin wrote in 1991 (*Ann Rheum Dis*; 50: 522-5) that "The American
experience with quality-assurance programmes prompted a Committee of the
Institute of Medicine of the National Academy of Sciences to conclude that for
Medicare recipients 'the current system is in general not very effective and may have
various unintended consequences' [ref.]. The Canadian system has similar roots but
to date has avoided some of the excesses of the American system. This paper traces
the growth and contrasts the system of quality assurance in America and Canada."

In the summary of their essay, those authors wrote that "America's system [of quality-assurance programs] is pluralistic, administratively very complex (and expensive!). In contrast, Canada's system is smaller in size, less expensive, and run by doctors. Both are increasingly preoccupied with 'bottom line' and with linking quality to cost containment efforts." They pointed out that "no one argues [i.e., questions] that health care can be improved and that a portion of the expenditure devoted to health care should be used to evaluate how we are doing," adding that "the costs of the system and the responsibilities of the system must be examined carefully . . ."

In 1992, "A survey of medical quality assurance programs in Ontario hospitals" was published by B. Barrable (*CMAJ*; 146:153-60). It was predicated on this: "It is generally believed that in recent years fewer hospital medical staffs have been undertaking quality assurance activities. ... Several reasons have been suggested for this, including but not limited to the following five:

- Confidentiality and fear of liability . . .
- A lack of compensation for physicians who involve themselves in quality assurance activities in addition to their regular clinical workload. . . .
- A loss of uniqueness and ownership. . . . [The quality assurance standards of the Canadian Council of Health Facilities Association, adduced in 1983] were very prescriptive about how medical staffs should conduct quality assurance. Before [1983] these activities were referred to as medical audits and were the exclusive domain of physicians [ref.]
- A dearth of expertise in conducting quality assurance activities. . . .
- The absence of comprehensive and clear legislation to encourage and, indeed, mandate practical approaches to medical quality assurance. . . . "

The survey questionnaire was sent to "The person deemed by the chief executive officer ... to be most responsible for medical administration," in "All teaching, community, chronic care, rehabilitation and psychiatric hospitals that were members of the Ontario Hospital Association as of May 1992." "Of the 245 member hospitals, participants from 179 (73%) responded, "indicating" a wide variety of quality assurance activities." Most common was that "In-hospital deaths were reviewed in 157 (88%) of the hospitals."

The legislature of Ontario introduced, in 2010, *An Act Respecting the Care Provided by Health Care Organizations* (Bill 46), amending or repealing various previous laws. This law stipulates that "Every health care organization shall establish and maintain a quality committee for the health care organization." This committee is to monitor the quality of the services and report on this to the responsible body, "with reference to appropriate data." It also is to make recommendations and to ensure that suitable materials on "best practices" are supplied to the care providers. Every healthcare organization also is to carry out surveys of consumer and provider satisfaction (annually and biennially, respectively).

This law, which calls itself the *Excellent Care for All Act, 2010*, mandates the quality committee "To oversee the preparation of annual quality improvement plans." These "must contain, at a minimum, (a) annual performance improvement targets; (b) information concerning the manner in and the extent to which health care organization executive compensation is linked to achievement of those targets; and (c) anything else provided for in the regulations."

In the city of Ottawa (in Ontario) in 2011, one such plan was published (as required) by the Montfort Hospital (http://www.hopitalmontfort.com/QualityImprovementPlan.cfm). The plan is:

- "to ensure that at least 65% of employees use proper hand hygiene before initial patient contact by March 31, 2012"
- "By March 31, 2012, achieve a substantial reduction in post-operative infection rate for abdominal hysterectomies . . ."
- "In collaboration with our partners, reduce the number of days that patients must wait for an alternate level of care (ALC) from 18% to 16.7%, . . ."
- "Reduce the wait times in the Emergency Department by 10% for patients with complex conditions and admitted patients . . ."
- "Increase the percentage of patients who would 'recommend the hospital to their friends and family from 73.9% to 85% . . ."
- [Etc.]

To each stated objective is attached the statement of how it will be achieved.

For the Ottawa Hospital, the corresponding QIP (http://www.hopitalottawa.on.ca/wps/wcm/connect/3870600046545f60a990fd2940f23d1f/QIP_short-e.pdf?MOD=AJPERES) is orientationally described by this Overview:

The Ottawa Hospital (TOH) aims to become a top North American hospital in terms of quality and safety of patient care. To this end, our Quality Improvement Plan (QIP) enhances hand hygiene and decreases the rates of hospital acquired infections. It improves effectiveness by avoiding preventable deaths and unnecessary readmissions, and continues our record of a balanced budget. It ensures patients are placed in the appropriate care setting when they no longer need acute care. Those who need care will see reduced wait times in Emergency. These actions will increase patient satisfaction and the quality and safety of care.

And its Ideas for Improvement are these:

- Monitor adherence to established best practice guidelines for central line infections, ventilator associated pneumonias, and medication reconciliation at discharge.
- Reduce Emergency Room overload through initiatives geared to reducing inpatient occupancy rates, including improving patient flow and reducing the number and length of stay of alternate level of care patients.
- Using champions and physician leads to promote hand hygiene as well as encouraging patients to ask staff to wash their hands.
- Use innovative ways to assess and improve patient satisfaction.

The foregoing, with its focus on Canada's Ontario province and the nation's capital city Ottawa in it, is instructive of the principal segment of public-health practice in the modern framework in which clinical medicine is public healthcare consequent to the advent of national health insurance.

The very first lesson from those facts is this: The Ontarian society, as the third-party payer of clinical healthcare, wishes to be assured that the societally sponsored care is of good quality, not only medically but economically as well. An expression of this is the very name of Ontario's Bill 46: Excellent [*sic*] Care for All [*sic*] Act (cf. above). In the Preamble of that Act, the first one of the nine brief statements about "The people of Ontario and their Government" is that they "Believe in the importance of our system of publicly funded health care services and the need to ensure its future so that all Ontarians, today and tomorrow, can continue to receive high quality health care."

Next to this belongs the lesson that the Ontarian people and their provincial government actually do not believe that all Ontarians now have, or in the future will have, high-quality healthcare: for, the government of the province is now mandating Quality Improvement [*sic*] Plans to be periodically developed and published by all of the province's hospitals (cf. above).

Third and most important, the province's government evidently presumes to be competent to tell the hospitals' personnel *how* the quality of care in them can and must be improved: it specifies the generic nature, though not the genesis, of those Quality Improvement Plans it requires.

It deserves note here that just before the Excellent Care for All Act was introduced, the province's Ministry of Health and Long-term Care called attention to "opportunities for improvement" (http://www.health.gov.on.ca/en/ms/ecfa/pro/legislation/ecfa_presentation_20100503.pdf). In Ontario (population about 13 million), it said,

- Forty thousand patients were admitted to hospital last year for ambulatory care sensitive conditions that could have been better managed in the community
- Last year, there were 140,000 cases of patients readmitted to hospitals within 30 days of original discharge
- Over 5,000 x-rays and 49,000 electrocardiograms were performed last year for patients about to undergo cataract surgery, when evidence shows these tests to have no clinical benefit
- Many Ontarians with diabetes and other chronic diseases are still not receiving all care recommended by clinical guidelines

Related to this is an instructional point of particular note: None of these substandard practices could have been identified – let alone remedied – by earlier implementation of such Quality Improvement Plans as have now been adduced (examples above) pursuant to the Excellent Care for All Act. The implication is that, while the hospitals are failing in their endogenous quality assurance, the government, in turn, is failing in its endeavor to provide "support to help them plan for and improve the quality of the care they deliver based on the best available scientific evidence" (quote, again, from the Act's Preamble).

The industry of hospital-based healthcare in Ottawa (and elsewhere) is quite anomalous among service (and manufacturing) industries at large: the hospitals lack built-in, serious *programs of industrial quality control*, in which the foundation of everything else is continual, *comprehensive monitoring* of the quality.

For any given hospital, we suggest, this would be a matter of continual, fair sampling of patients' stays in the hospital; abstraction of the records of the sample stays to form corresponding narratives of these, suitable for quality assessment; and periodic (monthly, say) evaluation of these representative narratives by the hospital's *quality review committee*. The quality assessments would focus on the broad topics of admission, diagnoses, treatments, adverse events, and discharge. They would focus on identification of deviations from 'community standards' (unspecified) and, especially, from specified 'guidelines' and 'best practices,' apart from addressing adverse events.

Periodically, typically annually, the evaluative findings would be summarized in terms of rates for the various types of substandard practice and adverse health event. These findings would be reported to the Chief Executive Officer (physician) of the hospital, for consideration and possible remedial action.

Any given hospital would need, for its serious program of quality control (normal in any commercial service-industry while missing in government-financed hospitals), *protocols* for the translation of hospital records into the corresponding narratives; for the documentation of the evaluative judgements; and for the reporting of these in terms of rates – all this with the understanding that these protocols need to evolve over time, as experience with them accrues and practices change.

As the development of these protocols would be contemplated in a given hospital in Ontario, it would be realized that the challenges, quite considerable, would be the very same in other hospitals in the same category of hospitals in the province, general hospitals, for example. Upon this realization, the interest in any given hospital would be in province-level development of the needed protocols, insofar as the hospital leadership and other professionals in the hospital indeed are interested in serious quality assurance for the care provided by the hospital. The interest would be in this protocol development by suitable representatives of the relevant set of hospitals, not representatives of the government of the province. (In Canada, healthcare is provincial, not federal, in its societal policy promulgation and administration.)

Thinking about the province-level development of protocols for in-hospital quality assessment, the planners in any given type of hospital would realize that there is considerable overlap in the nature of the programs across the different types of hospital in the province; that there really is a need for a single province-level *Agency for Quality Assessment*, with separate departments within it for each of the different types of hospital. Development of the quality assessment protocols would be the initial – and one continual – mission of this AQA.

This AQA would work with the hospitals' internal *clinical epidemiology units*. The CEU of any given hospital would sample the hospital stays, produce the case narratives from the records on each hospital stay in the samples, produce the periodic (annual?) statistical QA reports based on the QA committee's evaluations, and it would submit these reports to the hospital's CEO (cf. above). Another recipient of these hospital-specific QA reports would be the provincial AQA, which would collate them across all of the hospitals of a given type. The AQA would produce for each hospital the counterpart of the hospital's own QA report, concerning the aggregate of all of the other hospitals of the same type, providing this to the hospital. In addition, the AQA would produce, from each cycle of QA, an overall report for the Ministry of Health and Long-term Care.

The provincial AQA and the CEUs of the province's hospitals would, of course, be financed by the provincial Ministry of Health and Long-term Care, separately from the rest of the disbursements to the hospitals.

No introduction into industrial quality assessment and the rest of a production's quality assurance – in this instance in the service industry of hospital-based healthcare – is complete without at least a passing reference to the statistician who became the outstanding pioneer and authority on this: *W. E. Deming*. Quality of production to him was the production's *cost-effectiveness*, just as it is to a modern Minister of Health. We direct the reader to http://en.wikipedia.org/wiki/W._Edwards_Deming and through this to Deming's writings on the subject.

Regarding the need for quality assessment and assurance specifically in modern clinical healthcare, very instructive, in many ways, is John Wennberg's *Tracking Medicine: A Researcher's Quest to Understand Health Care* (2010). He notes that "even among the select few academic medical centers that reside at the very top in terms of their national reputation for excellence, there is little evidence that clinical practice is based on scientific consensus on the best way to practice medicine" (p. 170). In fact, he points to a variety of evidence to the contrary.

And finally, as for quality assurance in modern public-health practice, a supplement to the major innovation we suggested in the foregoing (cf. Preface) is a critical commentary from the wider industrial perspective, given in Appendix 5.

Appendix 1: Canadian Task Force on Preventive Health Care

> [Science] knows nothing of policy or utility,
> of better or worse.
> Torsten Vebler, 1906

> The scientist [has] neither the moral competence nor the moral right
> to use the lecture-room or the learned journal
> to pronounce *what ought to be done*.
> Max Weber, 1918

> Science never tells a man how he should act;
> it merely shows how a man must act
> if he wants to attain definite ends.
> Ludvig von Mises, 1963

> The Issue Advocate seeks to compel a particular decision,
> while an Honest Broker of Policy Alternatives seeks
> to enable the freedom of choice by a decision-maker.
> Roger A. Pielke, Jr., 2007

The first two of those here highly-relevant, orientational quotes above we drew from an indirect source, *The Scientific Life: A Moral History of a Late Modern Vocation* (2008) by Steven Shapin. He also cites three notable definitions of *vocation* right up-front, none of them consistent with the self-proclaimed mission of the CFTPHC (below).

As epidemiological research inherently is in the service of the practice of community medicine, and as this practice – epidemiological – is community-level preventive medicine, it is educational for a student of this research to gain familiarity with the Canadian Task Force on Preventive Health Care. Two sources of information about it are (refs. 1, 2):

O.S. Miettinen and I. Karp, *Epidemiological Research: An Introduction*,
DOI 10.1007/978-94-007-4537-7, © Springer Science+Business Media Dordrecht 2012

References:
1. http://canadiantaskforce.ca
2. Canadian Task Force on Preventive Health Care. Procedure Manual.
http://www.ualberta.ca/~mtonelli/manual.pdf.

"The [CTFPHC], previously known as the Canadian Task Force on Periodic Health Examination was established in ... 1976 by the Conference of Deputy Ministers of Health of the ten Canadian provinces. ... The particular characteristic that distinguishes the Task Force methodology from traditional approaches in decision-making on prevention issues is that *evidence takes precedence over consensus*. ... In the 1980s the Task Force methodology was adopted ... by the United States Preventive Services Task Force ... [both of them] developing *guidelines* for *clinical practice* and *public health policy*. ... In 2005, the [CTFPHC] was disbanded. In 2010 [it] has been established with the support of [Public Health Agency of Canada] and a renewed commitment and vision to continue its 25-year *tradition of excellence*." (Ref. 1; italics ours).

The CTFPHC is (ref. 2, p. 7) "an independent panel composed primarily of clinicians and methodologists that makes recommendations for clinical preventive actions ... but its work is also directly relevant to other health care professionals, developers of preventive programs, policy makers and Canadian citizens. ... The services must be provided in primary care settings or available by primary care referral."

"The CTFPHC uses the same definition of primary care as the US Institute of Medicine" (ref. 2, p. 36):

Primary care is the provision of integrated, accessible health care services by clinicians who are accountable for addressing a large majority of personal health care needs, developing a sustained partnership with patients, and practicing in the context of family and community. This definition acknowledges the importance of the patient clinician relationship as facilitated and augmented by teams and integrated delivery systems.

The CTFPHC is "an independent body of fifteen primary care and prevention experts who recognize and support the need for evidence informed preventive activities in primary care in Canada" (ref. 1). This body of experts is now chaired by a physician who is "a nephrologist, clinician-scientist and Associate Professor [in a Department of Medicine]" (ref. 1).

Having just been re-established, "The Task Force met in early 2010 to establish topic priorities and have begun the guideline development process. Topics being worked on in 2011 are:

– Screening for breast cancer
– Screening for hypertension
– Screening for depression
– Screening for diabetes
– Screening for cervical cancer
– Screening for obesity
– Screening for child obesity"

(ref. 1).

The CTFPHC classifies its recommendations as either "strong" or "weak." In addition to "the quality of supporting evidence," this classification is "influenced by

– the balance between desirable and undesirable effects;
– the variability or uncertainty in values and preferences of citizens; and
– whether or not the intervention represents a wise use of resources"

(ref. 1). A strong recommendation, either for or against an "intervention," is one in the context of which the Task Force is "confident" that its desirable effects "outweigh" the undesirable ones or vice versa. Weak recommendation corresponds to this outweighing being only probable in the judgement of the Task Force. (Ref. 1.)

It thus remains unclear whether individuals' values and society's interest in cost-effectiveness actually bear on the recommendations. The example in Appendix 2 strongly suggests that they don't.

So, the CTFPHC, continuing its "tradition of excellence," still seems to be about "periodic health examinations" rather than "preventive health care," though with the meaning of those examinations narrowed down to "screening." And as will be evident from Appendix 2 below, the meaning of screening, too, is narrower than it might be expected to be: rather than all of that which is involved in the pursuit of latent-stage diagnosis (rule-in), it is narrowed down to the initial test in this pursuit (in the diagnostic algorithm) – even though the recommendations are directed to clinicians rather than community doctors. And most remarkably, that diagnostic test is taken to represent "intervention" and thus to have "desirable and undesirable effects" instead of being, merely, a source of information.

Regarding such a test – for example, mammography on a woman with no overt indication of having breast cancer, or weighing (?) a child with no overt indication of being obese (!) – the CTFPHC approaches decision-making about its use with a "methodology" in which "evidence takes precedence over consensus" and evidence presents itself with a given level of "quality" but not quantity. The essence of this methodology, in its bypassing of consensus, remains a mystery, however. It is illustrated in Appendix 2 below.

Appendix 2: CTFPHC on Screening for Breast Cancer

Drawing further from reference 1 in Appendix 1 above, there is this piece of news:

> November 21, 2011 – The Canadian Task Force for Preventive Health Care has released an updated guideline for breast cancer screening in average risk women aged 40–74 … The new guideline, which *weighs the potential harms* of false positives and unnecessary biopsies *against the potential benefits* … updates prior guidelines by the Task Force from 1991 and 2001. (Italics ours; cf. App. 1 above.)

And there is also the guideline itself, separately for ages 40–49, 50–69, and 70–74, specifically in respect to mammography (as distinct from MRI and clinical breast examination). For this "intervention" the full specification is "mammography (film or digital) every 2 to 3 years." Everything about the guideline is contained on a single page.

For those three ranges of age the respective Recommendations are: "not routinely screening," "routinely screening," and "routinely screening." Each of these is characterized as "weak," the first two on the ground of "moderate quality evidence," the third based on "low quality evidence." (For the meaning of "weak," see App. 1 above.)

The Basis of Recommendation is specified, separately, for each of those three ranges of age. As an example, all that is said in reference to the age range 70–74 is this:

> Women who do not place a high value on a small reduction in breast cancer mortality and are concerned about false positive results of mammography and overdiagnosis may decline screening. About 480 women aged 70–74 die of breast cancer in Canada each year.

Associated with that Recommendation and that Basis of it is this declaration:

> To save one life from breast cancer over about 11 years in this age group [70–74],
>
> - about 450 women would need to be screened every 2–3 years
> - 11 women would have an unnecessary breast biopsy
> - about 96 women will have a false positive mammogram leading to unnecessary anxiety and follow-up testing.

O.S. Miettinen and I. Karp, *Epidemiological Research: An Introduction*,
DOI 10.1007/978-94-007-4537-7, © Springer Science+Business Media Dordrecht 2012

Besides, as for this range of age, "For every 1,000 women *screened for about 11 years*, about 5 women will unnecessarily undergo surgery for breast cancer" (italics ours).

To us it is very unclear what it is that thus is being said – and really meant – in respect to Canadian (*sic*; App. 1) women 70–74 years of age (who are "without personal or family history of breast cancer, without known BRCA 1 or 2 mutation, or prior chest wall radiation"). How can the option to "decline screening" be a "basis for recommendation" for screening? How can the annual number (*sic*) of breast-cancer deaths within this lustrum of age be a basis for recommendation about screening within this same, narrow range of age? or is it that at issue actually is *initiation* of screening in the early 1970s of age? And when said is that "To save one life from breast cancer over about 11 years in this age group [of 5 years], about 450 women would need to be screened every 2 to 3 years," is this about periodic screening in the early 1970s or "over about 11 years" starting in the early 1970s? And is that statement about one averted death "over about 11 years" a statement about the duration of screening or about the time horizon for the averted death or both?

That statement about "every 1,000 women screened for about 11 years" presumably is about women in whom the screening is initiated in the early 1970s of age. Thus it presumably is about screening that could be continued up to age 86 or so. But: "No data from our review addresses the benefits of screening in women … older than 74," implying that at issue actually is screening in the early 1970s only, for up to 5 years, and not "for about 11 years" starting at that age.

While the obfuscation in this guideline/recommendation statement is severe to the point of suggesting, to us, that it is intentional, *science writers* for newspapers evidently captured a simple message:

Five days after the publication of these guidelines/recommendations, a national newspaper of Canada (The Globe and Mail) announced, in a very prominent headline, that "Provinces re-evaluate breast screening." The subheading read: "Health-care providers are taking a fresh look at their rules and the costs of administering them." The article proper, by Renata D'Alesio, was about how those guidelines from the CPTFHC "have sparked a fiery national debate over which women should receive x-rays and how often."

In that same issue of that paper, another eminent headline read, "Cures for cancer at any cost"; and the associated subheading was, "The benefits of breast and prostate screening have been proved exaggerated, but we are no less invested in them." The author, Margaret Wente, ascribed that exaggeration idea to a statement, in 2009, by the chief medical officer of the American Cancer Society. Wente said that "The backlash [to the exaggeration idea] was ferocious. … The whole drama was repeated in Canada this week, …. The value of mammography screening, especially for younger women, has been decisively disproven. Many experts say it is of no value. Period."

One week after these articles, a headline in the same newspaper read, "When emotion prevails over cold, hard science." The subheading was, "Exceptionalism helps explain why mass breast cancer screening persists despite evidence it does more harm than good." The author, John Allemang, like his two predecessors (above), wrote as though he fully understood what the Task Force was saying. So he presented a very clear chart with the opening predicate: "If 2,100 women, 40–49, at average risk of breast cancer were screened every 2 years for 11 years." In it he presented the consequent numbers of cases of harm, while only "1 woman would escape a breast-cancer death," all of this pictorially illustrated.

The harms obviously would be incurred in the course of those 11 years, but what about the deaths that would be averted? By any reasonable presumption, the bulk of them would have occurred *after* that 11-year period of screening. Allemang did not indicate his understanding of what the Task Force meant in this regard, notably whether its time horizon for deaths was limited to those 11 years of screening; nor did he comment on his understanding of the relevance of the statistic that "About 470 women aged 40–49 die of breast cancer in Canada each year," being that 11-year screening initiated at age 49 presumably bears on deaths in the 1970s, even. He wrote about what he saw as the implications of "cold, hard science" when the Task Force itself based its recommendations on "moderate quality evidence" and "low quality evidence" (cf. above).

As we, different from science writers for popular press, have difficulties in understanding what the Task Force is saying about screening for breast cancer, and as "The particular characteristic that distinguishes the Task Force methodology from traditional approaches in decision making on prevention issues is that evidence takes precedence over consensus" (App. 1 above), we took a look at the evidence that was used. This the Task Force specifies in the *Canadian Medical Association Journal* 2011; 183: 1991-2001.

We found that two of the seven trials used as the sources of evidence enrolled women in the 70–74 range of age. In these, the total number of women of this age assigned to the screening arm of the trials the CTFPHC reported to be 10,339, but based on the trial reports themselves we found it to be $10,339 + 296 = 10,635$. The rest of the numbers are to the effect that the CTFPHC focused on the larger one of those experiences.

In this trial's report the *duration of screening* on women aged 70–74 at its initiation is not given in the original report; but according to the PDQ website of the NCI (of the U.S.), its duration was 3 years, not "about 11 years." The typical *duration of follow-up* (from entry into the trial) was 13 years overall but unspecified for those entering in the early 1970s of age.

The rates of death from breast cancer in the two subcohorts ($N_1 = 10,339$, $N_0 = 7,307$) evidently were derived, simply, as $49/10,339$ and $50/7,307$, their difference being $2.10/1,000$, not $2.22/1,000$. The "number needed to screen," as defined (App. 1), thus was $1,000/2.10 = 480$, not 450, at issue being screening for three (rather than about 11) years and death from breast cancer within 13 years (rather than ever). This 480 is but the statistical 'point estimate' from evidence so imprecise – as a matter of quantity rather than "quality" of the evidence – that the null P-value (one-sided) for the rate difference (and rate ratio) is as large as 0.04, and derived from a study in which the "Risk of bias," according to the CTFPHC, was "serious" – even with no regard for the incompleteness of the adherence to the regimens in the trial's two arms.

The Task Force drew the evidence for the three ranges of age solely from seven randomized trials, evidently believing that these indeed represent the useful segment of the research, of the entirety of it. At the core of this belief is the idea – highly aberrant – that the initial test in screening is an intervention, together with the associated idea – common – that an intervention's intended effect is to be studied by means of a randomized trial.

Such is the CTFPHC's reverence of randomization in the continuation of its "tradition of excellence" that it seemingly takes no notice of the quality-relevant particulars of this, while others see a sequence of embarrassments in this regard.

In his cancer-focused *The Emperor of All Maladies* (2010), Siddhartha Mukherjee relates some of the sad stories. In the Health Insurance Plan trial in New York, the entries into the study cohorts, randomly separated as to intention-to-screen, were initially without any determination/confirmation of the asymptomatic status, the women in the control arm of the trial not even knowing of their involvement in the trial; and later, women who were symptomatic on entry were removed from the index cohort, but they could not be removed from the reference cohort (p. 297). "Edinburgh was a disaster. ... [Various irregularities by both the doctors and the patients] confounded any meaningful interpretation of the study as a whole" (p. 298). And the nature of the randomization "completely undid the Canadian trial" (p. 298–9).

So here we have gained some insight into the Task Force working with its "renewed commitment and vision to continue its 25-year tradition of excellence" in which a distinguishing characteristic is that "evidence takes precedence over consensus" (App. 1). We see that this group makes authoritarian declarations of the form of knowledge (present or future tense) but with content that in principle is formed by mere results of studies, even very "low quality evidence" in this limited meaning of 'evidence'; and what is much more, those declarations can be grossly counterfactual about the studies' actual results. It is with this *pseudo-knowledge* as the principal input that the CTFPHC engages in its main mission: the *faux pas* (App. 1) of formulating authoritarian guidelines/recommendations for the practice of healthcare – clinical care.

Evidence per se, especially when misinterpreted (sect. 13.3) and seriously misrepresented, should *not* take precedence over consensus-seeking deliberations among genuine experts on a given topic of the knowledge-base of preventive healthcare (sect. 13.5) – of what is correctly understood to be preventive healthcare (see below).

Given what the CTFPHC says about its work in a general way (App. 1) and what it now says about screening for breast cancer specifically (above), and given also what science writers say about those new recommendations/guidelines (above), some additional critical comments are in order – for the student to "weigh and consider" (F. Bacon, sect. 1.4):

1. The CTFPHC classifies screening for a cancer (i.a.) as a matter of *preventive* medicine, invoking the concept of "secondary prevention" and saying that this is (by its own definition; ref. 2 in App. 1, p. 7) "directed to asymptomatic individuals with risk factors for a condition or preclinical disease (but not clinically evident disease)." But: our dictionary of medicine (Dorland's, 28th edn.) defines preventive as "serving to prevent the occurrence of," and preventive medicine, accordingly, as "that branch of study and practice which aims at the prevention of disease and promotion of health." Secondary it defines as "second or inferior in order of time, place, or importance; derived from or consequent to a primary event or thing."

2. The CTFPHC treats diagnostic testing, such as mammography, as an *intervention*. But: according to our medical dictionary (above), intervention is: "1. the act or fact of interfering so as to modify. 2. specifically, any measure whose purpose is to improve health or alter the course of a disease." Mammography is but a type of initial testing in the pursuit of early, latent-stage detection of – rule-in of diagnosis about – breast cancer. Instead of an effect (in terms of improvement in the course of the cancer), its yield is *information* (about the latent presence of breast cancer). The associated intervention – potential only – is the cancer's early treatment (in lieu of its alternative, late treatment upon the cancer already being overt, clinically manifest, symptomatic).

3. As the CTFPHC takes the *purpose* of mammography on asymptomatic women to be well exemplified by the concern "To save one life from breast cancer over about 11 years" and declares how many women "need to be screened every 2 to 3 years" to accomplish this, it leaves altogether unspecified the protocol/algorithm of the diagnostics-cum-treatment in each of those rounds of mammography; and the rest of the meaning also is obscure, to say the least (cf. above).

4. The meaning of this is not much clarified by the Procedure Manual of the CTFPHC (ref. 2 in App. 1). Said there (p. 36) is this:

> Evidence tables are also prepared, reporting information related to the key questions, the grade of evidence and the results. The Number Needed to Screen (NNS) is also calculated and added to the evidence table. NNS is calculated using the relative risk method: first a weighted relative risk (RR) must be calculated and then the number of lives saved per million ((1 – RR) multiplied by control group event rate per million) is calculated. Finally, the number needed to screen (1,000,000/lives saved per million) is calculated. ... All calculations and presentation of data in the evidence set are rounded to four [sic] decimal places.

5. While we had great difficulty understanding what the CTFPHC is now saying about screening for breast cancer and actually found the purportedly evidence-based statements to be seriously misleading about the evidence, and while the primary-care doctors receiving its Recommendations on screening for breast cancer likely are equally uncertain about what is meant, women do understand what a *given round* of screening for breast cancer is about: detecting and treating, at this time, a latent case of breast cancer, should a detectable case be present at this time – this with a view to the thus-enhanced prospects of *cure*

of the cancer. The word "cure" is in the title of Ms Wente's column prompted by the recent CTFPHC report (cf. above) while no reference to this concern is made in that report.

6. The following should be agreeable by anyone seriously concerned with the *intended* consequences of mammographic screening for breast cancer:

   – There is to be a definition, for a *given round* of the screening, of the *diagnostic algorithm* in all relevant respects (all the way to the rule-in diagnosis following biopsy); and this is to be supplemented with definition of the *treatment algorithm* following the cancer's rule-in diagnosis.

   – In reference to these regimens, the doctor's, rational *concern is to know*, specifically for the woman at issue, at the time: (a) the probability that a single round of application of the defined diagnostic algorithm would result in rule-in diagnosis of the cancer's presence; (b) the probability that the possibly detected cancer actually would be a life-threatening one; (c) the probability that the (possibly detected) cancer, if indeed life-threatening, would be curable by the defined early treatment while being incurable by any available late treatment; and (d) the time to the death that thus might be averted (ideally the probability distribution of this time, conditional on otherwise surviving).

   These concerns are in sharp contrast to the CTFPHC's "key question": "Does screening with mammography ... decrease mortality from breast cancer ... ?"

7. As for the *unintended*, harmful consequences of such a defined single round of diagnostics and potential early treatment, the concern is to know, again for the woman at issue, at the time, the probabilities of: (a) positive result (as defined by the algorithm) of the initial mammography (nothing "false" about this so long as a correct algorithm is correctly followed); (b) biopsy resulting from the work-up following positive mammography (nothing "unnecessary" about this so long as, again, ...); and (c) being treated for a cancer that actually is not life-threatening (cf. part 'b' above, the treatment in these cases, too, being necessary per the calculated risks accounted for in the protocol).

8. Even if all of this (nos. 6 and 7 above) be known from clinical (*sic*) research, unknown from research would remain the *valuations* that the particular woman at issue, at the time, associates with the probability of getting an already extant, latent case of otherwise fatal cancer cured by early treatment and with the probabilities of harms from the processes involved. All that the woman's realistic doctor can possibly hope to provide is that scientific knowledge input to the decision. The woman herself brings the valuations and, then, integrates these two sets of inputs – informally – into a decision about (the round of) the screening at the time.

9. If the CTFPHC would understand the nature of the requisite knowledge-base for rational decisions about mammographic screening for breast cancer, it would realize that *the relevant research remains essentially non-existent*. While it should understand its proper mission to be the formulation of the requisite

knowledge – experts' consensus – alone (à la IARC; sect. 13.5), in the prevailing absence of the requisite knowledge it has a particularly compelling imperative to refrain from putting forward purportedly research-based recommendations for practice. And even if the scientific knowledge be there, it should understand that "[Science] knows nothing of policy or utility, of better or worse" (App. 1).

10. The CTFPHC, after having studied this Appendix, should also study Appendix 3 below and then *reconsider* its "renewed commitment and vision to continue its 25-year tradition of excellence" (App. 1).

11. The Public Health Agency of Canada (of which the CTFPHC is part; App. 1) should be clear on whether it still – in this era of national health insurance – upholds its 'social contract' in respect to medicine, continuing to respect the profession's autonomy and limiting its public policies about, for example, screening for an illness to matters of cost reimbursement and its consequent concern for cost containment consistent with medically good-quality care (sect. 14.5).

Appendix 3: Needed Task Forces on Preventive Healthcare

Healthcare aimed at prevention of illness should be maximally *scientific* – not in the meaning of science telling doctors what to do (App. 1) but as a matter of having a rational theoretical framework together with knowledge-base from science. Preventive healthcare, when scientific, is directed to removal of known causes of illness (constitutional, environmental, and/or behavioral) or else to known ways to protect against their adverse effects on health. Scientific healthcare is *knowledge-based* – rather than 'evidence-based' – healthcare, with the understanding that the relevant knowledge is but part of the relevant inputs into decisions about preventive action.

While prevention-oriented health research abounds, it tends not to naturally translate into advancement of prevention-relevant knowledge (largely, we suggest, because of the prevailing nature of the scientific journalism surrounding medicine; sect. 13.6). There thus is a need for '*task forces*' with the missions to seek *to formulate the scientific knowledge* for the multifarious sectors of preventive healthcare.

Paradigmatic to these task forces can be taken to be the International Agency for Cancer Research within the WHO. Even when focusing on a given substance as a possible carcinogen, it makes elaborate ad-hoc arrangements in forming *topic-specific expert committees*; and these, then, work very seriously in the pursuit of consensus opinions (expressly refraining from making policy recommendations for practice; sect. 13.5). Paradigmatic is not only the ad-hoc formulation of narrowly focused expert panels, this by an agency that itself is no slouch in these matters. Of major note also is the fact that the IARC does not form Canadian and U.S. panels, or Scandinavian and Russian ones. It understands that scientific issues are *not country-specific but universal*. It is, after all, an agency of the WHO. (All members of the CTFPHC are Canadian.)

So, in the framework of the WHO – or some other global organization concerned with preventive healthcare – there should be a number – large number – of task forces in the meaning of differentiated *standing committees* for preventive

O.S. Miettinen and I. Karp, *Epidemiological Research: An Introduction*,
DOI 10.1007/978-94-007-4537-7, © Springer Science+Business Media Dordrecht 2012

healthcare. These task forces would not formulate their own consensus opinions on various topics; they would arrange suitable *ad-hoc panels* of even more differentiated, ultimate experts to do this.

One rather obvious example of these task forces would be that focused on radiation effects on health. It would arrange one expert committee to address the health implications of the use of mobile phones; another one focusing on the safety of the body scannings taking place at airports; and a third one on the health hazards attendant to medical imagings (incl. in screenings for cancers); etc.

The very multifarious topic of nutrition as a determinant of health would obviously require expertise very different from that having to do with radiation as a health hazard. In this centrally important area, at least two separate task forces would be needed, as the issues are so different between macro- and micronutrients.

In the formation of these, and other, task forces, one overarching principle is the one already insinuated by these examples: they should be *differentiated according to the respective determinants* they focus on, with no restriction on the health outcomes of concern. There thus should not be a task force for preventive cardiology, another for preventive oncology, etc. And there should not be separate task forces according to the recipients of the knowledge – general practitioners and community-level educators, for example.

À la IARC, the product from each expert panel should indeed be knowledge, not guidelines/recommendations. For, "Science never tells a man how he should act; ..." (App. 1).

Related to all this, we'd like to propose, for good measure, one task force of a very different kind. The various expert panels focusing on their respective areas of prevention-relevant research would have a shared problem: they would need to pursue consensus essentially through their intra-panel discourse alone, given the paucity of *public discourse* on the evidence per se for one, and on inference from evidence for another (sect. 13.6). So, a useful purpose would be served by an undifferentiated, single Task Force on Prevention-oriented Science, making recommendations on how to improve the journalism environment of this enormously important segment of health science (cf. sect. 13.6).

Appendix 4: On Introductory Teaching of Scholars

K.S. Miettinen

An adequate introduction into a scholarly field might prepare the student for further studies, and perhaps for initial steps in practice; but an excellent introduction is more ambitious: it establishes the foundations needed for a career, perhaps half a century in duration, and it specifically plants, at the beginning of that career, those seeds which may, with suitable experience and reflection, mature into wisdom by the time of retirement. A sign of an excellent introductory text is that the student repeatedly returns to it, cherishes it, and continues to deepen his understanding of it throughout his career. As D'Alembert put it, "To completely understand the elements [of a science] requires more than simply knowing what they contain. One must also know their use, applications and consequences. ... The distinctive trait of a good book about elements is leaving much to think about."

In reviewing numerous cherished introductions on my technical bookshelf, a number of common characteristics stand out: the best introductions motivate the field, clarify concepts, establish methodology (perhaps abstracted from progression of method), identify points of divergence from and convergence with related fields, warn the student about logical and conceptual problems, and recommend approaches for prudently navigating those problems.

An example of excellent introductory texts is Linus Pauling's "General Chemistry," a text which has stood the test of time (since 1947) and changed how chemistry is taught, specifically in introductory courses. The text motivates chemistry by depicting the universe as being composed of matter and radiant energy; weaves an exposition of scientific methodology into the sequence of chapters in an incremental fashion; explains difficult concepts such as temperature with precision; and identifies points of divergence from and convergence with physics.

The present introduction into epidemiological research has these same qualities, as it moves from grappling with the essence of the field to the knowledge that has been achieved; clarifies important concepts such as the study base; and identifies points of convergence with and divergence from related fields such as statistics and sociology.

O.S. Miettinen and I. Karp, *Epidemiological Research: An Introduction*,   171
DOI 10.1007/978-94-007-4537-7, © Springer Science+Business Media Dordrecht 2012

Points of divergence and convergence are often unknown to those who learn their field after it has reached steady state. For instance, a student searches in vain through modern introductions into logic for the reason why logic was reformulated in early twentieth century, or where modern logic diverges from classical logic. But fortunately, Alfred Tarski's "Introduction to Logic and to the Methodology of Deductive Sciences" is still available. Tarski explains the revolution in logic in terms of establishing the foundations of mathematics (and deductive science more generally), and throughout the text he points out the corresponding simplifications (e.g., neglect of the logic of properties – a matter of meanings – as distinct from the logic of classes, properties being unnecessary for establishing foundations of mathematics). Tarski is a case in point of what W. Edwards Deming repetitively emphasized, that "teaching of beginners should be done by a master, not by a hack," because so much of excellent introductory teaching consists of establishing nuanced understanding of fundamentals. An implication of masters teaching introductory courses is that these courses should generally have the highest students-to-teacher ratios, as beginners are the most common kind of student and masters the least common kind of teacher.

Tarski's inside knowledge also includes recognition of something that Deming never pointed out, namely that among masters we should prefer those of that generation which participated in the most recent revolution in the field.

This introduction into epidemiological research presents the insights of a seminal participant in the most recent revolution in the field, the theory innovations of the 1970s. In this transition to developing introductory material the senior author follows in the footsteps of scholars such as Andrei Kolmogorov, who famously toward the end of his career chose to focus on publishing introductory texts, developing a new state program of education in mathematics, and teaching introductory courses to young elite students in the belief that cultivating mastery of fundamentals in the next generation of mathematicians was the most valuable contribution he could make.

All fields of scholarly study have logical and conceptual problems; only the most dogmatic (and least enlightened) teachers would present their field as being problem-free. For instance, among the conceptual problems in mathematics are the semantic problem of what particular numbers (such as "3") mean, and the ontological problem of what infinity is. The solution of this in modern mathematics, via deployment of the abstract method, is to banish meanings of numbers as leading to too many fallacies; numbers are defined by the rules they follow without otherwise having any specific meaning. A good introduction (such as that of Timothy Gowers) tells the student that "for every number A apart from 0 there is a number C such that $AC = 1$" is a rule (the rule of multiplicative inverses), and that this is a rule for which zero is not an exception; it has no exceptions. Since the rules of arithmetic have no exceptions (else following the rules wouldn't sufficiently define numbers) and infinity does not conform to the rules of arithmetic, infinity is not a number. Such are among the first conceptual problems that a student of mathematics should be introduced to; there are many others.

Logical problems in a science generally are of two kinds: problems within the field, and problems about the field. In mathematics, for instance, a good introduction would familiarize the student with Goldbach's conjecture (a simple unproven apparent truth) and Wiles' proof of Fermat's last theorem (how can we know it is a proof?), as well as Skolem's paradox (do we understand what a real number is?). Such problems do not need to be solved for the student to have a successful career in a field, but understanding their difficulty is effective inoculation against professional hubris.

Poor introductions, by contrast, misrepresent the field at issue through dangerous simplifications that may make delivering the content to the student easier, but at the risk of misleading the student as to truth. For instance, in one introduction into statistics I read that "the objective of statistics is to make an inference about a population based on information contained in a sample and to provide an associated measure of goodness for the inference." This is, of course, a simplification that allows development of a mathematical body of statistical theory, but as a statement of objectives it is false in general, though perhaps true in special cases (such as opinion polling).

A better introduction into statistics would warn the student that this simplification, which undergirds the theory, is generally false, and that the general objective is to make inferences based on samples that can be validly applied beyond the population of which the sample is representative. For instance, the objective of the Framingham Heart Study surely was not limited to learning about the 1948 population of the town of Framingham. Going as far as is reasonable to validate inference from past data to future experience (a special form of the problem of inference to unsampled populations) without dogmatically reifying a metaphysical "state of nature" is the topic of Walter Shewhart's parvum opus "Statistical Method from the Viewpoint of Quality Control," a cherished introduction that I routinely reread. (Shewhart also addresses the more ambitious question of what evidence for the existence of a state of nature would look like; and as both Shewhart and his most prominent apostle Deming point out, all rigorous attempts to develop evidence indicating the existence of a state of nature have failed.)

Whereas all scholarly fields have logical problems, a good introduction explains those problems while demonstrating valid ways to navigate them. For example, Athanasios Papoulis' classic introduction into "Probability, Random Variables, and Stochastic Processes" opens with a chapter on the logical difficulties with the very concept of probability (independence of the axioms and the various definitions), which leads to demonstration of how comparing the quantum mechanical theories of Maxwell/Boltzmann, Bose/Einstein, and Fermi/Dirac requires using three definitions of probability in a three-stage process. The classical (a priori) definition is used to develop quantum mechanical models, the axiomatic definition is implicit in the theory of probability with which the models are manipulated, and the relative frequency definition is used in empirical testing of the model predictions. The logical problem of developing the theory of probability is exposed to the student rather than concealed, and prudent handling of the resulting difficulties is then demonstrated.

The present introduction to epidemiological research gives the student similar exposure to logical difficulties with what now are held as standard epidemiological methods (such as cohort and case-control studies), and presents their needed corrections.

Should any child of mine choose a career in epidemiological or related research I would look forward to their being taught from this text, by one of the authors or some other master, with the hope that the youngster would be a fertile receptor and career-long cultivator of the wisdom sown here.

Appendix 5: Quality Assurance for Modern Public-health Practice

K.S. Miettinen

I welcome the request (see Acknowledgements) to bring the perspective of industrial quality control at large to bear on what in this text is suggested for the industry of hospital-based healthcare (sect. 14.5). While agreeing with the suggestions in this text, I add some philosophically relevant background to motivate and augment the call to action.

The statistical and epistemological methods of W. Edwards Deming (originally of Walter Shewhart, Deming's teacher) are central to modern industrial quality control, service industries included. The first two of his famous 14 points for management are: "Create constancy of purpose toward improvement" and "Adopt the new philosophy."

Deming explained in his writings that while various stakeholders in an enterprise may have different interests – a labor representative may be concerned with employee morale and job security, investors and taxpayers with costs, consumer advocates with customer satisfaction, etc. – all of these concerns are interrelated, and regardless of which one is valued, the appropriate plan of action focuses, solely and constantly, on improvement of quality.

Thus, the pursuit of quality is an indirect means of pursuing myriad other things, which may or may not be publicly stated objectives. This is reflected in the observation in the present text that good healthcare is not only medically good but also economically good, that improving the medical quality of care is a way to indirectly pursue also other societal objectives related to healthcare.

In nominally pursuing improved quality, as Deming explained, we should really pursue greater uniformity of the goods produced or of the services provided. This point is rooted, first, in his insight that the causes of poor quality are also causes of variation in quality, so that effective pursuit of better quality and effective pursuit of more uniform quality are identical. And besides, he pointed out that while a rigorous epistemological basis for defining the limit to how far we can go exists for uniformity, it often does not exist for excellence. Thus, quality improvement should be pursued indirectly in terms of reduction in variation.

O.S. Miettinen and I. Karp, *Epidemiological Research: An Introduction*, 175
DOI 10.1007/978-94-007-4537-7, © Springer Science+Business Media Dordrecht 2012

Finally, in nominally pursuing greater uniformity (lesser variation) of quality we should really pursue greater randomness of variation in quality. This point is rooted in his insight that a system whose variation of quality satisfies rigorous tests for randomness is unimprovable, no matter how broad the variation in quality happens to be; such a system can be replaced or redesigned, but its operation as designed is as good as can be achieved. On the other hand, a system whose variation of quality exhibits signs of nonrandomness can be improved by locating and removing the causes of nonrandom variation, no matter how narrow the range of variation already is. Greater uniformity too must be pursued indirectly, by eliminating nonrandomness rather than by directly addressing the variation.

Thus, industrial quality improvement à la Deming consists of two activities: continuous effort to identify assignable causes of variation in systems whose results show statistical evidence of nonrandomness, and regular redesign or replacement of systems apparently operating with only random variation. A notable implication of this is that while there may be acceptable levels of absolute quality and/or of variation of quality for some purposes, there is no acceptable level of either of these for the purposes of quality control. This is because, as I noted above, industrial quality control is an indirect means to achieving numerous other objectives (e.g., cost reduction), rather than just quality per se.

This insight of Deming's is the basis of his exhortation to eliminate management by objective: there is no rational basis for setting a standard for what is acceptable. What is needed is constant pursuit of improvement, whatever be the level of performance already achieved.

Thus, in the quality improvement plan for Montfort Hospital cited in the text, the problem with the plan to ensure 65% compliance with handwashing protocols is not the absurdly low level of the goal; it is the very idea that an acceptable level can be rationally assigned. The plan should be to identify and eliminate assignable causes of variation in handwashing practices; and when that has been driven to the extreme of apparently no remaining assignable causes, then the follow-on plan should be to rethink and redesign workflows so that further improvements in the rate of handwashing can be made. Redesign of a system that is not yet in control is contraindicated; much of the information and insight that is needed to design a better system is not available until the existing system truly is operating as it was designed to operate.

The approach outlined in the text, involving sampling-based monitoring of care processes (rather than outcomes), is directly analogous to the sampling-based monitoring of processes currently used in other industrial programs of continuous improvement. I would add that in the industrial programs in general the information from samples is not used to identify causes of variation; it is used, instead, to indicate when it would be economical to initiate inquiry into causes of the variation. For the process of searching for assignable causes of variation costs time, money, lost productivity, and often also pride and workplace harmony. For these reasons, such inquiries are kept to a minimum. Statistical sampling of processes (not merely records; the sampling should produce data not otherwise recorded) provides the basis for deciding when to search, and it limits the scope of where to search and what to search for; but the identification of an assignable cause of variation (an object of repair, retraining, or disciplinary action) is never made on the basis of the sampled data, it is made only on the basis of a thorough inquiry triggered by statistical anomalies in the sample data.

There are details of Deming's perspective that would lead to augmentations of the quality assessment program sketched in section 14.5 beyond sampling of the records by sampling of the processes to produce new data. Some of these may be worth mentioning. In the text the authors proposed review, by an in-hospital panel, of narratives of the care of individual patients. This is, no doubt, salutary, and representative of the activities of development programs in all professions But the Deming perspective is not to focus on the sequence of processes that a unit (e.g., a patient) passes through, but rather focus on the sequence of units that pass through an identifiable process (e.g., colonoscopy). Both perspectives provide valuable information, but it is the latter perspective that enables the statistical search for evidence indicating nonrandom variation.

The rates of untoward findings should not be the basis for remedial action as suggested in the text: Deming often made the point that rates themselves do not communicate whether a system is operating at capacity. Instead, they provide raw material which epidemiologists would be well qualified to critically examine in searching for evidence of performance levels outside of system control limits. Epidemiologists would provide this service by combining rates of untoward findings with other facility-specific information, for example on demographics of the served population, caseload during the period in question, experience level of staff, etc., to assess whether an observed rate of untoward findings deviates enough from experience across other facilities to warrant an inquiry into the existence of assignable causes of variation at that facility.

These details of a program of quality improvement can be worked out once hospital administrators become acquainted with and adopt the conceptual framework of continuous improvement. There will, however, be institutional obstacles to adopting this framework, which need to be thought through. Deming's industrial quality improvement philosophy requires close collaboration among the parties involved in ways that differ from models of confidentiality and proprietary information currently fashionable in medicine. In manufacturing-related industrial settings, part of the means to avoid expensive inspections of purchased goods (e.g., parts purchased from a supplier for further assembly) is the requirement that vendors provide evidence of quality control of their processes along with their deliveries, so that purchasers can confirm that a lot of goods was produced under suitably controlled circumstances; the goods themselves are not inspected; instead, information about the vendor's internal processes is disclosed along with the delivery. In a hospital setting, the analogue would be providing to those concerned, patients included, a report on the degree of uniformity achieved in the processes relevant to the quality of the provided care.

Even though medical institutions are supposed to be self-policing, it is not enough to supply quality-assessment reports to the hospitals' quality-assurance boards and government regulators, for these entities are not interested in the quality in the classical sense of the term. They do not have a stake in the quality of care, as they do not suffer the consequences of poor-quality care. While the persons in those functions may well have the best interests of patients and society at heart, management practices are generally anchored to the interests associated with the positions involved, rather than to presumptive virtues of the people assigned to those positions. Society at large, and patients in particular, have a stake in the quality of healthcare, so they are the genuinely interested parties to whom evidence of internal quality control should ultimately be disclosed.

Administrators and regulators have a two-tiered responsibility in quality control: first, to drive the continuous pursuit of quality within systems operating as designed, and second, to rationally redesign systems operating at the limits of their capacity for better performance. It is with respect to the first of these two that assurance of performance should be provided to patients and to society at large, and it deserves note that this is not information of a professionally esoteric kind; information about the state of control of internal processes is largely non-technical and thereby comprehensible to the general public. This information does not tell patients whether their specific care will be (or was) good or not, but it can assure them that the systems that care for them are operating at capacity, that is, that the care being provided is statistically as good as can be reasonably expected of the system. On the other hand, information supporting redesign of workflows should be shared within competent professional communities, notably among administrators of similar facilities across the jurisdiction involved.

The application to medicine of the quality control methods of industry at large is complicated by the fact that medicine is a service industry (not unlike, e.g., the hospitality industry). Even though the methods pioneered in manufacturing have been successfully applied in service industries as well, banking and hotels being outstanding examples, many problems specific to service industry have been identified in these applications.

One of the most difficult problems in service industries in general is that enterprises tend to serve captive audiences; there is little pressure from distant competitors, and therefore considerable difficulty in motivating the necessary constancy of purpose necessary for continuous improvement. In line with this, there are rarely two general hospitals operating across the street from one another, and hospitals at a distance are only slightly in competition with one another.

Another problem of service industries is that they do not face elastic market demand; a service enterprise cannot expand the overall volume of business in its segment (e.g., by productivity breakthroughs that lower costs); it can at best take market share from competitors. Thus, a hospital that lowers the cost of delivering babies may take business away from other hospitals, but it is unlikely to affect the overall number of births in a given population. Improvements in the cost of child birth are not rewarded with a baby boom.

In service industries there is a tendency to sample users of the of service regarding their satisfaction, while really needed for quality control is sampling of the processes that go into providing service. Just as quality control in manufacturing cannot be based on examining finished products, so also quality control in medicine cannot be based on interviews of served recipients of care. Medical care in larger institutional settings provides opportunities for sampling of care processes, while the service processes of solo practitioners are difficult or impossible to document.

A final problem typical of service industries, and shared by medicine, is the problem of one-of-a-kind in service environments. No two hospitals have the same layout, or serve demographically identical populations, or have identical average ambulance transportation times from residential neighborhoods. As a consequence, each facility is likely to implement distinct processes, and therefore lessons learned at one facility may not be transferrable to another, and rates of error will be difficult to compare between facilities. Some service enterprises, chain restaurants and some hotel chains being prominent examples, have made great efforts to standardize facility layout and location (e.g., relative to road intersections) in order to mitigate the one-of-a-kind effect, and the results have been truly remarkable. Many diners may not think of chain restaurant food as being of 'high quality,' but when quality is understood in terms of eliminating nonrandom sources of variation, then it is indeed of very high quality – it is very consistently what management specifies it should be, the diners' wishes notwithstanding. The degree to which such standardization is possible (or politically acceptable) in medicine remains to be seen.

As medicine shares with certain other service industries (e.g., education) the peculiar structure of having third-party payers cover some or most of the expense, this structure poses certain further challenges for quality assurance, notably agency conflicts and data quality (objectivity) challenges. Whereas third-party payer systems are inherently prone to shift costs, that is, charge some customers more than the true cost of their service in order to subsidize similar service to others (e.g., cost transfers between urban and rural populations, or between wealthy and poor populations, etc.), third-party payer systems tend not to generate objective cost data on the services rendered – the subsidies are hidden in the cost data, making the data not truly representative of costs under management. Without reliable data, quality assurance is greatly complicated, if not precluded outright.

Where possible, the remedy would be to separate the subsidy function from the function of rendering service, for example by having the government restrict its role to paying subsidies (and monitoring regulatory compliance) and allowing the private sector to render service (and collect geographically varying market fees). Similar separation could be accomplished between national and state/provincial governments, to a degree. Such separation of duties is called for in all aspects of management practice where the integrity of data is a concern, and it is the management analogue of the principle of separation of powers in government, whereby preventing concentration of responsibility in one branch makes collusion, concealment, and deception more difficult. The argument for separation of duties is only indirectly an efficiency argument; it is directly a transparency and integrity argument. Separation of duties is an aspect of system design intended to expose information that might otherwise be concealed or distorted, by documenting the information in the public interactions of the separated parties. This information is then available for better management toward whatever objective is socially desirable, be that efficiency, equity, availability, or quality.

Major cultural changes are required if programs of improvement in hospital-based healthcare were to be brought to the standards of service industry in general, but this should not deter taking on the mission. One reason for setting out to meet the challenges is the enormous improvement not only in manufacturing but in service industries as well consequent to the introduction of the quality control ideas in the 1920s (the time of the original work of Shewhart, Dodge, and others). And another, burning reason is the well-known and ever worsening cost crisis of modern healthcare. The authors' gambit deserves both attention and follow-on.

Author Index

Subject Index

O.S. Miettinen and I. Karp, *Epidemiological Research: An Introduction*,
DOI 10.1007/978-94-007-4537-7, © Springer Science+Business Media Dordrecht 2012